Testimonials

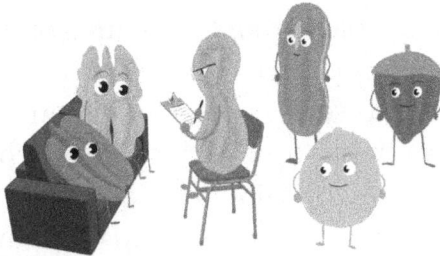

It is a great pleasure seeing in print the second of three books emerging from the insightful research of Dr Bronwyn Wilson. As the principal supervisor for Bronwyn's PhD, I witnessed the meticulous exploration of neurodiverse relationships that she undertook for this research. This book is not just a compilation of research findings but a compassionate resource for anyone connected to neurodiverse families and couples. Participants' voices are sensitively and faithfully represented throughout these pages, contributing to a more informed understanding of neurodiverse relationships. This makes the book a vital resource not just for therapists and service providers, but also for individuals and communities to raise awareness and foster greater inclusivity and a more empathetic world.

Dr Susan Main
Senior Lecturer | Academic Integrity Officer
School of Education | Edith Cowan University

Have We Gone Nuts?

Even though I have worked in this field for about thirty years, I loved how Bron brought all the understanding and research together in a fresh and particularly pertinent way. But more importantly – despite her studious research in working from a series of academic texts and papers, she has made this potentially scholastic topic of neurodiverse relationships utterly real and relevant in everyday language for ordinary lay-people – from the mouths of 400 participants who have this shared experience. Each chapter has food for those hungry to seek more about their relationships – whether they are in a couple relationship, whether they are in a relationship by extension such as a friendship, or even touching on professionals who need to know more about these relationships. Every professional should have a copy of this work, especially if they are in relationship counselling - to be more targeted, proactive and supportive with their skills honed in their work with neurodiverse clients. For all involved, this book is a plethora of useful information. But more importantly Bron, in this second book, has given increased voice to this oft ignored, misunderstood, sometimes written-off or even maligned group of people; she has given compassionate understanding to both the neurotypical and the neurodivergent (AS) parties; and she has given them an international presence and acknowledgement. Thank you Bron.

Dee Jones
Finding Solutions and Kamo Counselling

THROUGH THE WORDS OF 400 INTERNATIONAL
RESEARCH PARTICIPANTS

Have We Gone
Nuts?

The Family, Friend and Clinician's Guide to Neurodiverse (Autistic-Neurotypical) Relationships

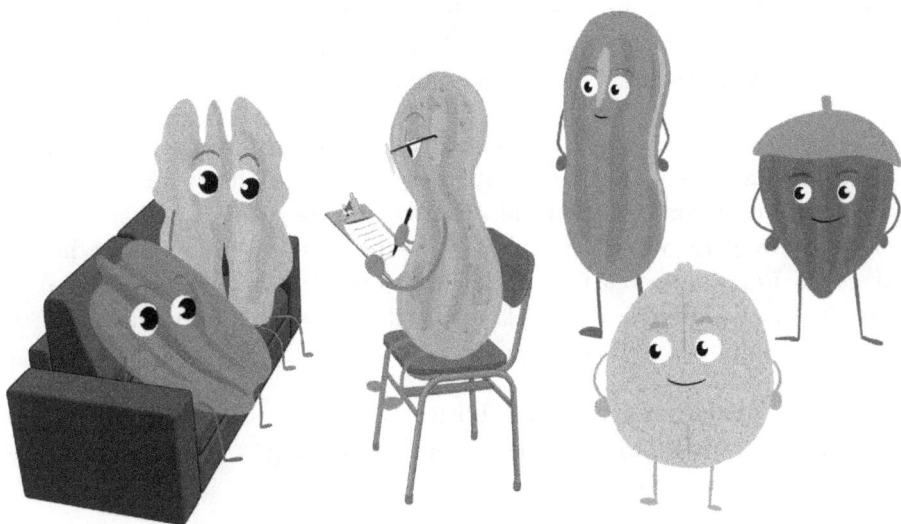

Dr Bronwyn Maree Wilson

Foreword by Professor Tony Attwood

First published by Ultimate World Publishing 2024
Copyright © 2024 Dr Bronwyn Wilson

ISBN

Paperback: 978-1-923123-58-8
Ebook: 978-1-923123-59-5

Cover design: Ultimate World Publishing
Layout and typesetting: Ultimate World Publishing
Editor: Marinda Wilkinson

Ultimate World Publishing
Diamond Creek,
Victoria Australia 3089
www.writeabook.com.au

ULTIMATE WORLD
—— PUBLISHING ——

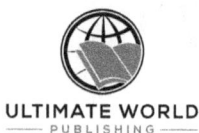

Dedication

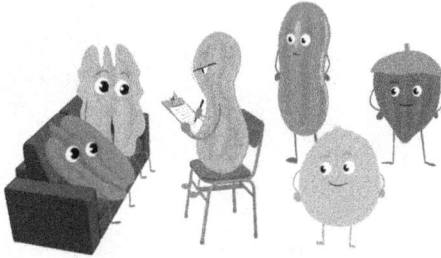

This book is dedicated to my husband Michael, who inspired me to return to further studies and continues to support and encourage me to devote time and attention to my research and writing.

I would also like to dedicate this book to my immediate and extended family members, who along with numerous friends, bestowed on me substantial understanding of the impacts of Autism Spectrum Conditions on and within relationships.

Contents

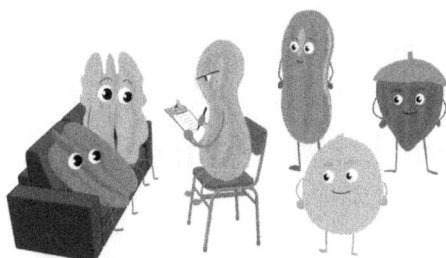

Contents

He placed me in a little cage,
Away from gardens fair.
But I must sing the sweetest songs
Because He placed me there.
Not beat my wings against the cage
If it's my Maker's will,
But raise my voice to heaven's gate
And sing the louder still!

Lettie B Cowman, Streams in the Desert

Foreword for
Have We Gone Nuts?

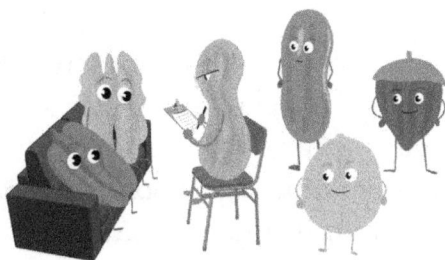

Autism has many qualities that can appeal to a potential
partner. These include honesty and integrity, kindness and
social naivety, an intense passion for their interests, and
a strong sense of social justice. There can be technical or
artistic abilities and good career prospects. The non-autistic
partner may recognise characteristics they are familiar with
in a parent, which leads to a natural understanding and
connection. The autistic individual's difficulties with social
situations can be perceived by their non-autistic partner as
awaiting their transformation through their social expertise
and extensive social network.

The early stages of dating may not indicate to either
partner the long-term relationship issues associated with

autism. The autistic partner may have camouflaged and suppressed their autistic characteristics to be more attractive to a non-autistic partner. They may have acquired a dating 'script' from watching romantic movies and created a 'mask' or artificial persona. However, eventually, the mask is removed, often when the relationship is formalised, and it becomes apparent that the autistic partner has difficulty with the intuitive understanding of how to maintain a long-term relationship.

Gradually, some of autism's characteristics can cause distress and conflict in the relationship, such as difficulty reading social cues, expressing feelings, the frequency of social experiences, emotion regulation and repair, expression of love and affection, intimacy, communication, conflict management and household responsibilities. These issues reflect many of the themes in conventional relationships, but autism can explain the reasons why these issues have become deeper and more resistant to change.

Some of the issues in the relationship can be due to aspects of 'Theory of Mind', a psychological term that describes the ability to read facial expressions, body language, tone of voice and social context to determine what someone is thinking or feeling. Both partners experience this. We have known for some decades that autism is associated with Theory of Mind difficulties, which are part of the diagnostic criteria. However, we now recognise that the non-autistic partner can also have trouble 'reading' the inner thoughts and feelings of their autistic partner. This is described as 'Double Empathy'. The autistic partner may not express subtle emotions in facial expressions, tone of voice, or body language that are easy for their partner to read.

Foreword for Have We Gone Nuts?

In a conversation, the autistic partner can struggle to find the words to express thoughts and feelings due to aspects of interoception and alexithymia. That is the sensory perception of the body signals that indicate emotional states such as heart rate and breathing (interoception) and being able to translate the emotions that you feel or remember into speech (alexithymia). This will affect the ability of the autistic person to disclose their inner world and communicate their feelings. As the relationship progresses, the non-autistic partner will anticipate increasing self-disclosure as a sign of the depth of the relationship and trust, not recognising a genuine difficulty in perceiving and communicating their inner world to their partner.

Autistic adults can achieve successful social engagement, but this may be by intellect rather than intuition. Thus, social occasions are mentally exhausting and energy-draining. In contrast, the non-autistic partner may find that social experiences require little mental energy and may create energy. The initial optimism that the autistic partner will gradually change and become more socially skilled and confident can dissolve into despair that social skills are static due to limited motivation and energy to be more sociable. The non-autistic partner may reluctantly agree to reduce the frequency and duration of social contact with family, friends and colleagues for the sake of the relationship. However, they feel deprived of experiences they enjoy and find refreshing rather than exhausting.

Although the couple lives together, the autistic partner has a diminishing need for social, conversational and leisure time together. The autistic partner can be content with their own company for long periods. Although the couple is living together, conversations may be few and primarily involve the exchange of information rather than enjoyment of each other's company, experiences and shared opinions.

Autism is associated with experiencing strong emotions, especially anxiety, anger and depression and difficulty coping with stress at work and home. There may be issues in the relationship regarding anxiety because the autistic partner can be very controlling, and life for the whole family is based on rigid routines and predictable events. There may be concerns regarding anger management and the risk of physical and psychological abuse, and both partners may be vulnerable to being depressed.

The non-autistic partner often expects emotional comfort to repair their distress, but gestures of love and affection may not be perceived by an autistic person as an automatic emotion repair mechanism, with a hug perceived as an uncomfortable squeeze which does not make them feel better. A typical comment of the non-autistic partner is that hugging their autistic partner is like 'hugging a piece of wood'. The person does not relax and enjoy such close physical proximity and touch.

The autistic partner can be accused of being callous, emotionally cold and lacking empathy. However, this is due to a genuine difficulty reading interpersonal signals and intuitively knowing how to respond. The non-autistic partner gradually realises that they need to be very clear and direct in expressing their feelings and suggesting to their partner what they need to do to repair their emotions, and as described in the previous book, *Have They Gone Nuts?* need to almost continually prompt the anticipated response.

Foreword for Have We Gone Nuts?

In a conventional relationship, regular expressions of love and affection are expected. A metaphor for the need and capacity for expressions of love and affection can be that a non-autistic partner has a 'bucket' capacity for love and affection that needs to be regularly filled and replenished. In contrast, an autistic partner has an affection 'cup' capacity that is quickly filled. The autistic partner may be perceived as not expressing sufficient affection to meet the needs of their partner, who feels affection-deprived and unloved, which can contribute to low self-esteem and depression.

I thoroughly enjoyed reading *Have We Gone Nuts?* especially the quotations from over 400 research participants. Bronwyn explains and illustrates our increasing awareness of how autism affects relationships, including both partners not perceiving and meeting each other's needs, difficulty explaining the relationship issues to friends, family and professionals, and the importance of increasing relationship counsellors' knowledge of how autism affects a relationship. As described on the cover, this book is written for couples, family members and clinicians. From my perspective as a clinician, it is written in an engaging and informative style, and I look forward to reading the next book in the series.

Professor Tony Attwood

Introduction

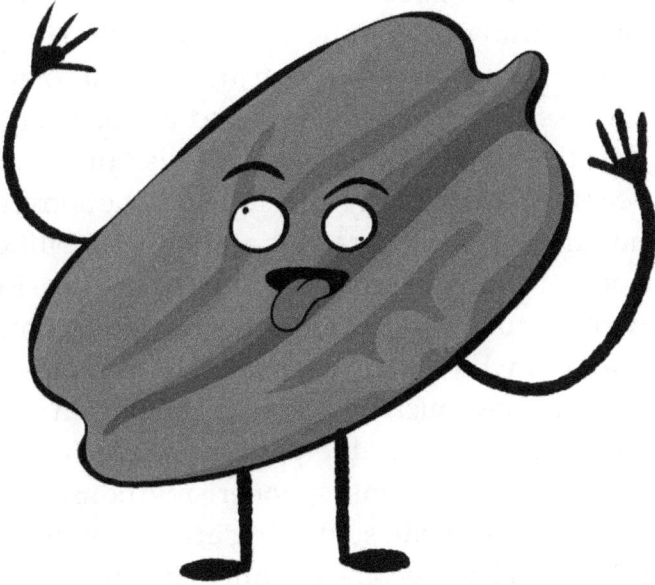

Crazy Making

Have We Gone Nuts?

'If you're going through hell, keep going.'
Winston Churchill

Legacy and Loss

My father was a kind and gentle soul who was always on the lookout for a good chat. Walking through town, he would often annoy my mother by repeatedly stopping to talk with this person and that. She just wanted to get there. His father was the epitome of a refined English gentleman, having left the United Kingdom with his family when he was 11 years old. Particularly talented with the spoken word, my grandfather's brilliant orations and MC capabilities were called upon at many events and important occasions. He certainly could turn a phrase. Both men were accomplished communicators who married capable and complex women who did not display much warmth. My mother, an intelligent woman who had a love of the patterns found in language, would often use neologisms, spoonerisms, nonsense words and puns for amusement, so playing around with language and word games had become a family custom.

Sadly, my grandfather suffered a stroke, which all but robbed him of his verbal abilities. Watching him struggle with the loss of his impressive speaking skills was heartbreaking. Later, when my father died, the family lost its soul. His no-nonsense stabilising influence was no more, and some parts of the family spun out of control. Although it is well known that complex emotions are experienced in the processes of grief and grieving (Stroebe et al., 2017), at one of the most distressing of times, I was to face some of the worst of human behaviour.

2

Crazy Making

I arrived home from university to find a collection of teenage boys painting an upturned bicycle with red spray paint in the middle of the kitchen floor. My sister and her teenage sons had moved in with me, not long after our father had died. With my teenage children, it was a house bursting at the seams. There had been a few challenging episodes, but this surpassed them all. It was a rental property. My name was on the lease. I was attending university to obtain a teaching degree, while also working part-time sewing curtains for a retail curtain store. Near to the painting misadventure was a pair of full drop curtains ready to go. The potential for disaster was obvious. I exploded at the boys to get that bike and paint outside! Why they had been spray-painting inside was beyond me. There was plenty of space for that outside. When she found out, my sister was not amused, to say the least. However, not at the boys – at me! How dare I yell at her boys! Well, that decided it. I took her out for a meal to soften the blow and told her that this situation was no longer going to work for me. She would need to find somewhere else to live. Then it began!

Day and night, I began to receive phone calls from people I did not know who would harass me, while questioning my mental capacities. Various family members became more and more convinced that I was mentally unstable. I did not understand. What was happening? I was working part time while completing a full-time university degree. Although money was tight, I was keeping food on the table and a roof over our heads. My teenage children had all the basics. Why had people suddenly begun doubting my reasoning? Bit by bit my life was becoming more frightening. As more and more people started hounding me, I felt that I was up against an invisible monster who was eating my life away. Protesting only seemed to strengthen the allegations of the accusers. 'People that are mentally unstable always deny that they are mentally unstable.'

The continual harassment ensnared me. I could not disagree. I could not agree. I was powerless. I started losing weight at an alarming rate. Friends became concerned. Phone calls persisted. The anonymous callers kept on badgering me. They continued to pass judgement on my rational functioning. Certain that I was experiencing mental challenges, many in my family began doubting everything I was saying. I decided there was only one thing left for me to do. Get away.

New Beginnings, New Explanations

After some time, I had been able to put that unpleasant chapter behind me. I was living in a different city, my studies completed, a new marriage, a full-time teaching career and my adult children within easy reach. Then, I made an astounding discovery. Embarking on this different way of life had not only rescued me from the most difficult of circumstances, it also led to finding out what lay beneath those circumstances.

My teaching career had awakened an understanding of the autism spectrum – along with a growing realisation that many of my immediate and extended family members were most probably on the spectrum. Armed with a desire to know more, I said goodbye to teaching and embarked on another new journey, this time into research. Entering teaching had activated what leaving teaching had crystallised. Born from years of reflecting on the details of challenging interactions, both inside and outside of the classroom environment, my research focus was on communication in neurodiverse (autistic-neurotypical) relationships.

To my surprise, apart from the main research findings, the process of undertaking research had given me an unexpected result. Not only did I gain understanding of the communication difficulties in neurodiverse relationships, but it also gave me an insight into my sister's behaviour. It made me realise just how my sister's retaliation had been able to accomplish its far-reaching influence over my life.

Individuals on the autism spectrum have difficulties with communicating. They are often very uncomfortable with change and have a strong need for predictability. Their black and white thinking also lends itself to narrow ideas about the way in which life should happen. My sister and I had made an agreement that we live together. To her, I was making a change that she was unprepared to accept. To her, I had gone back on my word. She did not tell me these things. I had only begun to realise this as my understanding of autism grew.

A shrewd person, my sister had known just how to concoct a cunning plan. Therefore, the situation we had found ourselves in was not merely a quarrel between sisters. And it had not ended at a dispute caused by miscommunication. It had become something much worse. Attwood (2015) explains that the feelings of anger for those on the spectrum can be extremely intense, often leading to explosive rage. My sister's intense rage had led her to the conflict resolution strategy of 'an eye for an eye'. When an injustice is perceived, Attwood (2015) reveals how those on the spectrum can use this 'eye for an eye' approach with the intent of inflicting at least equal, if not more, discomfort on another as a legitimate means to achieve what they presume as deserved justice.

However, perception does not always make something absolute. And while that reasoning may seem shocking and extreme to say the least, in my sister's mind she was inflicting on me what she saw as a justifiable punishment. I must suffer at her hand to compensate for the suffering that she perceived I had inflicted on her. And suffer I did!

Despite having reached somewhat of a resolution between us at a later stage, sharing my newfound realisations with her was not possible. She could not accept this renewed me. This more educated me. This me, who now had a voice. Who could speak with conviction and could stand my ground. Yet, simmering beneath my new life was a dark residual of that past. I only found out about that much later.

Two From Two

Have We Gone Nuts is the second book in a three-book set that describes the results of two research studies on communication within neurodiverse relationships, that is, relationships in which at least one person is on the autism spectrum. The two studies extended over a period of eight years, with the investigation of the second study based on the findings from the first. The broad focus of both studies was on adults with an autism spectrum condition (ASC) and communication in their close relationships. Particular attention was devoted to the characteristics of prompt dependency (a behaviour that can develop due to difficulties with self-reliant behaviour and self-initiation skills), accompanied by prompting (a behaviour used to persuade, encourage or remind a person to do or say something).

In the studies, 400 research participants describe the 'craziness' and yet, also 'not craziness' of living on the inside of a different kind of relationship. A relationship that looks quite 'normal' on the outside but is anything but on the inside. Conveyed from the distinct position of each group of participants, the three-book series is designed to be an informative journey behind the closed doors of neurodiverse relationships. The words and perspectives of adults with ASC, and those whose are neurotypical (NT), are interwoven together as we journey through the various topics under investigation in each book.

In the first book, the two behaviours of prompting and prompt dependency converging into a communication cycle was found to be caused by the very different needs of each person within these relationships with regards to emotional reciprocal interaction (that is, the need to avoid reciprocal interaction versus the need to have reciprocal interaction). The underlying dynamics of the prompt dependency cycle was illustrated by revealing how the elements of the cycle interacted within a complex system of competing needs, roles, expectations and problem-solving behaviours. In other words, the first book described all the internal relational aspects that are a consequence of this communication system and how it impacts on those within these relationships. Also provided were identifiable actions for people in neurodiverse relationships to consider implementing to encourage the potential to thrive.

Have We Gone Nuts?

Although it may be read in isolation, this book builds on the information contained in the first. Through the participants' narratives, we discover the different approaches to life between people on the autism spectrum and neurotypical people and how this affects their relationships. Also explored is what takes place when they reach out to family, friends and services from professionals, for comfort, validation, encouragement and support.

A persistent lack of research about autistic adults has hindered community recognition and understanding of how autism manifests in adults. This widespread lack of awareness is a factor in why many people worldwide fail to notice that autism may be a consideration for the people in their lives. The participants' reports highlight the difficulties that this lack of awareness creates for them. We learn about:

- The diplomatic balancing act that they are often required to perform when talking with family and friends about their ordeals
- The awkward situations they go through from the distorted interpretations and opinions that others often hold
- The unhelpful reactions, opinions and conclusions they regularly face
- The disbelief or dismissal of their version of events.

Equally, since many clinicians and counsellors went through their education at a time when the autism spectrum was relatively unknown, this book is intended as a resource to gain an understanding of the difference between neurodiverse relationships and typical relationships. Specific considerations covered are:

- The pairing of autistic and neurotypical people establishes particular relational nonconformities
- The exclusive unconventionality of neurodiverse relationships
- The reasons underpinning this unconventionality and the outcomes that result
- The features of this unconventionality that causes conventional therapies to be ineffectual.

For that reason, this book aims to enhance awareness of these matters as the participants share the challenges they face when involved in clinical settings and their viewpoints about the different approaches they need.

The last book in the series shares the research data. It will be crucial for policy makers, practitioners and other stakeholders to utilise the data from this study to inform program improvement and future program development.

So, who are the research participants? Firstly, a Master of Special Education research (a small-scale study of nine couples) was completed at Griffith University, Brisbane, Australia in 2013. The nine couples all comprised one person who was diagnosed or self-diagnosed with Asperger's Syndrome and one NT person. The Doctor of Philosophy research (a larger international study) followed two years later and was completed at Edith Cowan University, Perth, Australia in 2020. Included were partners, parents, adult siblings and adult children involved in neurodiverse relationships; specifically, relationships that include people with ASC and neurotypical people. Most participants were from Australia, the United Kingdom and the United States of America, with others from Africa, Asia, Canada, Europe, the Middle East and New

Zealand. To protect anonymity, all interview participants were assigned a pseudonym.

The *Have They Gone Nuts?* series is intended to be used as a resource for neurodiverse families and couples. It is for anyone who suspects they may be in a neurodiverse relationship; family and friends of people in neurodiverse relationships; counsellors, therapists and service providers who work with the neurodiverse population; those who research neurodiverse relationships; and anyone who wants to increase their understanding of neurodiverse families and couples. It is hoped that by sharing the thoughts and experiences of the 400 participants involved in the studies, it will not only promote greater understanding of this population, but will also assist in bridging the knowledge gap that currently exists between many service providers, the community in general, and those within or connected to neurodiverse families and couples.

1

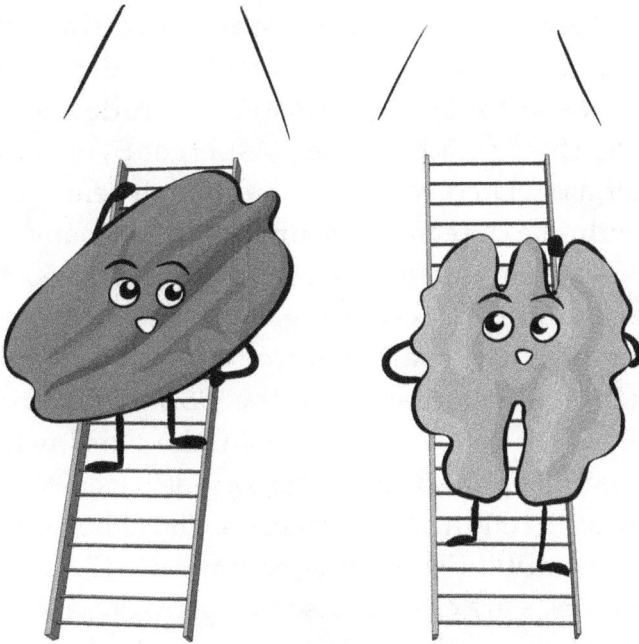

Climbing the
Awareness Ladder

Have We Gone Nuts?

'Life isn't about finding yourself.
Life is about creating yourself.'
George Bernard Shaw

The Evolution of Understanding

The autism spectrum, autism spectrum disorders (ASD), and more recently, autism spectrum conditions (ASC)[1] are terms used to describe various neurodevelopmental conditions that include autism, Asperger Syndrome (AS), and other associated conditions. Although referred to as a single syndrome, autism can be understood as many different conditions, with the common factors being biological, rather than behavioural (Casanova & Casanova, 2019). Despite this, diagnosis is usually centred on behaviour. Baron-Cohen (2015) states that while the *DSM-5* uses the term 'disorder' when referring to autism, the word is a legacy from an earlier period in the history of psychiatry and it may be time to rethink our categories. Thus, the term autism spectrum condition is gaining recognition (Baron-Cohen, 2015). The ASCs are characterised by early-onset difficulties in social communication and unusually restricted, repetitive behaviour and narrow interests. These characteristics impact

---

[1] ASC stands for autistic spectrum condition. This term is sometimes used by those outside the medical profession to describe someone with autism. Education and social care professionals have questioned whether autism should be viewed as a disability, as indicated by the word 'disorder' and that we should move away from the negative images associated with the term. The abbreviation ASC is becoming more widespread in use, especially in schools.

on the capability to do well within everyday interaction and consequently impact on the quality of life for those with ASC and those with whom they interact.

The present-day notion of autism has evolved significantly. Derived from the Greek for 'self', it signifies persons living in their own world rather than the world of others (Tantam, 2012). Early descriptions suggested that autism was the result of childhood psychoses or psychodynamic disturbances of parent-child relationships. This flawed belief gave way to advances in medical science, which have established autism to be a neurobiological condition of early brain development.

The term autism has only been in use for approximately 100 years. Its original use by a Swiss psychiatrist around 1911 referred to one group of symptoms of schizophrenia. However, autism existed long before it attracted a label. It is found worldwide, with considerable evidence to indicate its existence throughout human history (Deisinger, 2011). One of the earliest accounts was found in a 13th century book describing, the behaviour of a Franciscan monk indicative of a person with autism (Deisinger, 2011). It has been said that many famous historical figures would probably have been diagnosed with autism if they had lived today. Albert Einstein, Amadeus Mozart, Sir Isaac Newton, Charles Darwin and Michelangelo are among many who have exhibited considerable behaviours suggestive of autism (Elder & Thomas, 2006; James, 2005).

Generation Lost

Despite extensive steps forward in knowledge and understanding of autism, there are many unknowns regarding autism in adulthood. Research attention usually remains on children or on the biomedical aspects of autism (Lorant, 2011; Pellicano et al., 2014; Wainer et al., 2017). Very little research has been conducted on adults and even less has been conducted in relation to their close relationships. What little research has been accomplished has produced conflicting conclusions (Atherton et al., 2021; Sachdeva & Jones, 2018). To date, it remains unknown what proportion of autistic people manage to attain adequate levels of social integration as adults or how many experience a good psychological and physical quality of life (Howlin & Magiati, 2017).

When considering that community knowledge and attitudes usually emerge from discoveries made during research, and that many professionals went through their education at a time when autism was relatively unknown, few people have a concept of how autism manifests in adults. Since many professionals continue to have tunnel vision, focusing only on children when they discuss autism spectrum conditions, many people form impressions that autism is essentially a childhood difficulty. Countless people who ought to be diagnosed, reach adulthood without a diagnosis (Lehnhardt et al., 2013) and autistic adults, with or without a diagnosis, largely remain misunderstood. Even rudimentary understandings that the ASCs are lifelong conditions are seldom openly contemplated and practical solutions for adults, their family members, and others who provide support services are often neglected. Some people mistakenly think that childhood trauma is a trigger for autism to materialise in adulthood. The idea that autism is a permanent brain-wiring condition, that people do not grow out of their autism, and that an autistic child will become an autistic adult, is often not understood, or not given a lot of thought.

False impressions of autism in adulthood are also perpetuated by TV and social media and strengthened by performances that present autistic adults as easily recognisable; that autism manifests as either a genius with obvious autistic traits or a quirky likable nerd type who basically keeps to him or herself, also with recognisable characteristics. That a person can be on the autism spectrum without immediately obvious signs appears to be inconceivable to much of the general population. Many clinicians and counsellors, also unfamiliar with autism in adults, doubt that autism could be a possibility for their adult clients and, as a result, do not distinguish autistic features from diagnosed disorders with which they are more familiar (Lehnhardt et al., 2013).

With new frontiers of how females correspond, as well as heavily contested attitudes toward many aspects regarding autism, such as, autism's possible historical longevity, diagnostic criteria for autism and Asperger's Syndrome[2] (AS) (Tsai, 2013), what is, or is not part of the autism spectrum especially in adulthood, how autism should be evaluated, the specifics of language, descriptors and definitions people should use to describe autism, beliefs about female diagnosis

---

[2] Debate continues in the autism community regarding the dissolution of the AS label within the broader classification of ASD due to the higher functioning distinction. T. Attwood (personal communication, March 17, 2015) specified that although AS is now designated as ASD level 1 (Asperger's Syndrome) in the *DSM-5*, the term Asperger's Syndrome is still in transition in clinical settings and within the community and continues to be applied in these settings. For continuity and simplicity, and to respect the preference of people previously diagnosed with AS, the term *Asperger's Syndrome* will be used in this book.

and whether a diagnosis should even be a concern for adults are all issues that continue to be questioned and challenged. Not only do myths and falsehoods proliferate in these circumstances, but also, regularly, differences of opinion trigger worldwide hostility. These matters and antagonisms prevent consistency of opinions and understandings, especially across different countries. Is it any wonder that professionals and people in the community alike, struggle to understand autism in adults?

Consequently, and in view of the high variability to autism, this inadequate understanding of autism in adulthood has led to a widespread failure to recognise the needs of adults on the spectrum, the needs of their significant others and what's more, can often cause errors of judgement, mistakes in guidance and even the provision of incorrect approaches to therapy or support. Real harm can result. Frequently, this population are left marginalised, without professional or community support and without the support of family and friends.

Debates, Doubts and Diagnosis

Although Asperger's Syndrome (AS) is no longer recognised as a diagnosis in and of itself and is now part of the broader category of autism spectrum conditions, many still use the term. Individuals who would previously been identified with AS usually have average or above-average intelligence. Clinically, their features can look like those of schizophrenia, anxiety disorders, obsessive-compulsive disorder, avoidant personality disorder, attention deficit/hyperactivity disorder or personality disorders, and these similarities can lead to a failure to diagnose autism or to receive a misdiagnosis, especially in adulthood (Kosger et al., 2015). According to Lai and Baron-Cohen (2015), it is often only people with more severe symptoms, such as extreme social aloneness, no eye contact, and frequent motor mannerisms, or those with concurrent developmental difficulties, such as cognitive or language delay, who tend to receive a diagnosis prior to adulthood. Less noticeable people, such as those who would previously have been identified with AS and those with more subtle difficulties, tend not to be diagnosed until much later, if at all. Consequently, the lives of adults often remain a mystery, especially those who are misdiagnosed or undiagnosed. Yet it is those with more subtle difficulties who are more likely to be involved in a neurodiverse relationship, and therefore require the help and support of clinicians, together with the understanding and support that ought to be gained from family and friends, especially at times when the relationship hits problems, a frequent occurrence.

Additionally, while possessing the cognitive capacity to achieve well in life, those with less obvious difficulties often have proficient levels of language that operates alongside a failure to process the language of others (Edwards, 2008). Edwards (2008) specifies that 'the more sophisticated the person's language is, the greater the problem may be' since those on the spectrum frequently give 'a false impression of their comprehension … leading to much misunderstanding, confusion and stress' (p. 52). Not only do they have difficulty with interpersonal communication, but they also appear to prefer non-social experiences and need less social interaction when compared to the general population (Benning et al., 2016). Consequently, many extremely able adults with autism commonly struggle with day-to-day life skills. These difficulties and differences will more than likely lead to problems in relationships, and therefore, require specialised help and understanding from clinicians, counsellors, and family and friends.

Until recently, autism was thought to affect more males than females. While one explanation is the different gender socialisation patterns, and the different ways in which females deal with experiences (Attwood, 2007), another explanation is that females do not fit the behaviour profile of the male-oriented diagnostic criteria (Carpenter et al., 2019). Simone (2010) explains that 'women on the spectrum are a subculture within a subculture. We have many of the same quirks, challenges, habits, traits and outlooks as men, but with our own twist. It is not so much that Asperger's syndrome (AS) presents differently in girls and women, but that it is perceived differently, and therefore is often not recognised' (p. 13). Even when females on the spectrum are identified, they usually receive a diagnosis much later than equivalent males and also need to exhibit more severe autistic symptoms and greater cognitive and behavioural problems to meet the criteria (Bargiela et al., 2016).

Besides, females appear to be more skilled than males at using protective and compensatory factors, such as observational learning to interpret and imitate facial expressions, and creating scripts for social interaction, while applying rules by rote to social-emotional situations and friendships. These strategies can give the appearance of social conformity and integration with their peer group (Carpenter et al., 2019; Tierney et al., 2016). Since both males and females with autism frequently remain unidentified, unnoticed and unsupported, they face considerable personal, social and professional barriers to fulfilling their potential as intelligent and independent members of society. Their struggles with communication and interpersonal relating can limit their ability to form meaningful relationships (Baldwin et al., 2013) that may have devastating consequences for their social and mental wellbeing (Cooper et al., 2017). Equally, these limitations extend to the social and mental wellbeing of their significant others.

There is also a further argument which is gathering force. In the 1990s, the autistic self-advocacy movement emerged with the assertion that autism is a valid way of being. Sakellariadis (2011) explains that:

Although seemingly bizarre behaviours of people on the autistic spectrum are still considered pathological by some, current literature questions established boundaries of normality and suggests that autism is a condition better understood as one expression of the human condition (p. 1).

Leadbitter et al. (2021) agrees, stating that 'the growth of autistic self-advocacy and the neurodiversity movement has brought about new ethical, theoretical and ideological debates within autism theory, research and practice' (p. 1). The neurodiversity movement suggests that there is no standard brain, and in today's world we live in a 'disability culture', where all human beings exist along 'continuums of competence' (Armstrong, 2010, p. 3-11). However, den Houting (2019) argues that although the neurodiversity paradigm frames autism as a difference and a cultural identity, not a disability, people with autism are, very often, disabled. Adding to this notion, den Houting (2019) reports that while it could be the result of a failure of their environment to accommodate their needs, the considerable variation and fluctuation in both capability and capacity that people with autism experience needs to be considered. Further, considering autism to be both a natural variation and a disability, allows for support and services when needed, and also provides acceptance and respect for people with autism, as valuable members of society; a deficit-as-difference conception of autism (Kapp et al., 2013). Thus, the notion of autism, that was first considered a mental illness, and more recently an information processing problem, is still under development as we progress through to a more informed, sophisticated and nuanced understanding of the neurodiversity paradigm, by producing research that includes, rather than excludes, the voices of people on the autism spectrum (den Houting, 2019).

There are also strong convictions on both sides of the debate between the use of person-first language (e.g. 'person with autism') and identity-first language (e.g. 'autistic person') (Nicolaidis, 2019). While the American Psychological Association (APA) advocates the use of person-first language, the disability culture advocates the use of identity-first language (Dunn & Andrews, 2015). According to Shakes and Cashin (2019), the adoption of person-first language originates with the disability movement's attempts to reduce discrimination for people with a disability by placing significance on the person rather than their disability or health condition. On the other hand, attributed to the neurodiversity movement, the implementation of identity-first language has gained momentum within autistic advocacy associations and throughout literature with identified autistic authorship (Shakes & Cashin, 2019). Thus, the discourse of the autistic community, the widening of the autism spectrum and the establishment of the autistic self-advocacy movement has necessitated that appropriate and sensitive ways to refer to people's disabilities are considered (Bagatell, 2010).

However, the identity-first approach does present some language challenges in regard to communicating about disability. Shakes and Cashin (2019) make the point that 'word choice, labels and the like, whether written or spoken, become a challenge because it matters who is doing the representing, who is being represented, and with whom an exchange is occurring' (p. 260). Additionally, previous to the *DSM-5* changes to diagnostic criteria, receiving a diagnosis of Asperger's Syndrome was less associated with disability and dysfunction than was autism (Smith & Jones, 2020). The perception that society is autism-phobic and perceives autism as a significant disability whereas Asperger's carries the more positive stereotypes of being quirky, but likeable, has meant that even though it has formally ceased to exist, many still want to adopt the label of AS, as an identity (Smith & Jones, 2020). Therefore, identity-first language may be seen by some as undesirable, while others find it desirable. The study conducted by Shakes and Cashin (2019) found no identified research that systematically explored and considered antagonisms and potential consequences of either mode of language becoming dominant. In the absence of empirical studies to guide practice, it is important that language selection is based on context and the preference of the individual (Shakes & Cashin, 2019). To address the various preferences, these different representations will be used interchangeably throughout this series of books.

This overview of adults with autism presented above supplies the backdrop to the topics explored in this book. A prevalence study of the Centres for Disease Control early in

2022 confirmed that the majority (59%) of autistic individuals do not have an intellectual disability. These books are directed toward those who do not have an accompanying intellectual disability; to discuss the experiences of people involved in neurodiverse relationships, to provide insight into specific obstacles that they encounter, specifically when seeking help and support. While most of the participants involved in these studies discuss their romantic neurodiverse relationships, some also discuss their neurodiverse relationships with adult children, parents and siblings. So, let's meet the participants.

What a Difference a Diagnosis Makes

For adults, growing up in a time when autism was barely recognised, and then, receiving a diagnosis of autism later in life or becoming aware and self-diagnosing, they need to come to terms with the knowledge that they have unknowingly lived with the condition their whole life. This realisation can present some challenges to a person's self-concept, likely to be either a source of shock or one of relief (Stagg & Belcher, 2019). It can be just as profound for the neurotypical (NT) people in their lives. Each person will need to make sense of what it means for their lives as their awareness and understanding grows.

When asked if his diagnosis had changed things for him, Samuel (ASC) answered:

Absolutely, yes. It has changed my entire life … Yes, I simply do not want to do what is necessary in order to simply please her. It's too much of a struggle, it takes too much mental energy and I did that too much with my first wife and I started out doing it here but in knowing that I'm wired differently and in order to act normally is a real strain. I'd rather just save my energy and enjoy myself doing what I want because what I get back from Sally isn't enough to really want it. I'm getting enough of what I need here simply being looked after.

Beth (NT) described her husband's relief once he had received a diagnosis:

His diagnosis explains a lot of his behaviours and attitudes and because we were going to get divorced, we went to marriage counselling and he did some anger management courses as well, so he's done a lot of therapy ... Yes, yes, yes, he's very happy with it. Initially he wasn't, no he wasn't happy being hospitalised, that was the first hospitalisation, the second hospitalisation is when he got the diagnosis and then he said, 'Oh my God, my whole life has been explained by this diagnosis.'

An anonymous survey respondent (ASC) also described this relief:

Since the discovery I have of ASD, I feel I woke up from a coma, and now on a journey of healing of 65 years of not knowing this about myself.

On the other hand, Dana (NT) revealed how she was the one who felt relief:

I didn't want to say, you have Asperger's. I was really tempted to do it, but I was like 'Ooh it's you, it's you, it's you, it's you' ... but it was like I felt all this weight of all this. I mean 20 something years of all this exploration. Finally, just went Ahhh!! I get it! I get it! So, all of a sudden, I have a real direction. We had always thought for a long time that there was something and I knew it was a commonality between that family group because for years I've always thought 'none of you people are comfortable in your own skin'.

Mandy (NT) also felt encouraged that her husband's diagnosis had allowed some improvement in their discussions:

We went and got diagnosed so he understands it well now, so we can talk about it. Although we don't talk a lot about it now because he uses it as an excuse, but it's something that I'm able to express to him the frustration and why, and it's not having a go at him as much, it's just explaining that that's normal for him. I just have to learn to live with it.

Sometimes the diagnostic journey is a long tedious trek without finding answers until a child in the family receives a diagnosis. Rachelle (ASC) said that was the case for her:

It's hard to sort of define whether its seeking help for myself or my relationship or my every single other relationship that's sort of gone wrong ... I saw, it was in the 20s ... psychologists and psychiatrists and doctors and counsellors etc. etc. Trying to work out what was wrong and then finally my son was diagnosed and then I was diagnosed.

However, sometimes a diagnosis journey does not end with confirmation of autism but triggers further investigation and additional diagnoses. There is increasing evidence that autism is associated with other conditions such as attention deficit hyperactivity disorder, dyslexia, hyperlexia and other language disorders, together with intellectual disabilities, to name a few. Terry (ASC) described how learning about himself, becoming more aware of his conditions and talking it out with his family were helping him work towards improving his self-understanding:

I think I'm doing a lot better than I used to and being aware of the various conditions that I have, Asperger's diagnosis from about 6 or 7 years ago I think it was, and the problems I have with anxiety and PTSD from my service time, so … I did have the opportunity to talk to my sister about a few of these things and the way it is in the family and knowing that my older brother is obviously more on the spectrum than I am, or possibly that I've had more social interaction than he has and self-development of myself, or trying to in recent years. But yeah, talking about and looking at the other members of the family then talking about my father and his reluctance to communicate or show emotions and my older brother being very similar to that it seems to be the side of the family that has these particular traits and it was interesting and probably good for me to talk to my sister about it … yes it was positive.

On the other hand, sometimes the diagnostic journey for autism may start with an accurate diagnosis of another condition, such as an eating disorder, substance abuse, gender dysphoria, borderline personality disorder or other mental or personality disorders, which may later be followed by a diagnosis of autism. There is also an association between autism and Tourette's disorder, sleep disorders and bipolar disorders. Ultimately, there are many different ways to arrive at a diagnosis of autism. Consequently, clinicians and counsellors need to be aware that they may need to consider a diagnosis of autism and by doing so, adapt their methods to accommodate those who have different ways of perceiving, thinking, learning and relating compared to typical populations.

Support Thoughts

A diagnosis can make a substantial difference to the lives of those in neurodiverse relationships. Contributing to greater understanding of the particular difficulties, a diagnosis is especially valuable for those with more subtle difficulties such as those who previously would have been identified with AS. They are more likely to fly under the radar, but also, are more likely to establish relationships.

Potential benefits to receiving a diagnosis are:

Understanding
- The relief of having answers to feeling different
- An appreciation of diversity rather than feelings of 'abnormal' or 'alien'
- An explanation of past and current difficulties
- The ability to access appropriate information

Belonging
- Obtaining a sense of identity
- Obtaining self-acceptance among like-minded individuals
- Obtaining a right of entry into an alliance

Strategies
- Learning from others who fully understand the reality of living with neurological differences
- Learning from others about how to cope with difficulties

- Learning from others about how to cope with other people's lack of knowledge

Family
- A diagnosis can provide accurate understanding, tolerance, acceptance, modifications and empathetic responsiveness to and for the whole family.

Despite the many benefits of receiving a diagnosis, there are various reasons why a diagnosis may not be attainable for many adults. Obtaining a formal diagnosis is an expensive process. Often it is very difficult to access, especially from appropriately qualified professionals. Along with this, some adults come to an understanding of themselves and self-diagnose, usually after a child in the family has gone through the diagnostic process at school. Adult family members may then recognise their own similar characteristics and difficulties.

Also, since many neurodiverse families and couples present to a counselling or therapy session without an awareness of what may lay at the foundation of their difficulties, they and their therapist may not consider autism. Generalist training does not suffice to cover all variations of autism, and as a result, many professionals lack understanding that their clients may be on the autism spectrum, leading to overlooking this prospect. For diagnostic benefits to be realised, it is key that an increase in community and professional recognition of autism in adults is achieved so that a reconsideration of the way intervention strategies are conceptualised, devised and implemented can be established (Lorant, 2011).

Whether formally or informally diagnosed, awareness that autism is a contributing factor to the differences and difficulties experienced in a relationship is key to beginning the journey of discovery of what autism in adulthood means for the many neurodiverse relationships worldwide.

The following chapters take a deeper investigation into the differences between people on the spectrum and neurotypical people and what to take note of when contemplating whether the autism spectrum is a consideration for you or for people in your family, your friends or your clients.

2

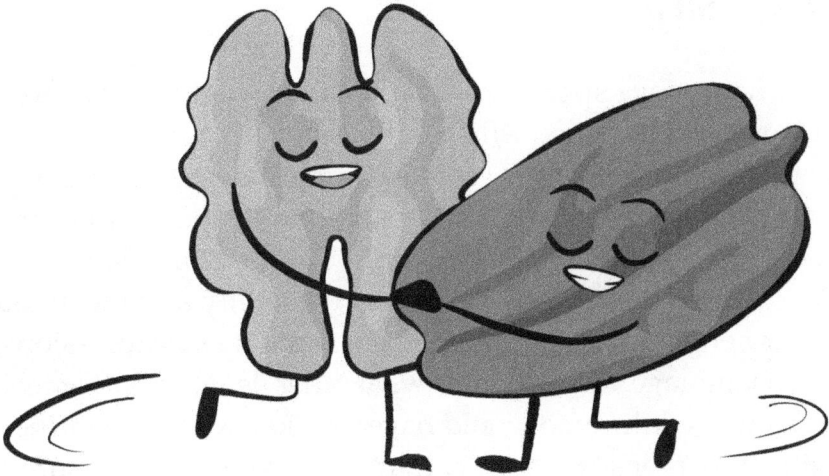

Dancing with Difference

Have We Gone Nuts?

**'We must not only learn to tolerate our
differences. We must welcome them as the
richness and diversity which can lead to true
intelligence.'**
Albert Einstein

Out of Step

The autism spectrum is a highly prevalent neurode-velopmental condition which is the result of a genetic variance in the hardwiring of the brain with significant differences in the anatomy and function of specific brain regions associated with social behaviour (Donovan & Basson, 2017; Sato et al., 2017). These brain variations affect the ability to understand other people as well as being able to read facial expressions, body language and also infer what other people think or feel. Although adults who would have previously been identified with Asperger's Syndrome, that is, those with more subtle difficulties, are less visible and less apparent than those with classic autism, it is misleading to think that the impact of autism is any less challenging for them or for those in their lives.

Due to the wiring of their brain, all people on the autism spectrum have one thing in common. With more subtle difficulties, or with more obvious signs of autism, diagnosed or not, with more complications or not, with comorbidities or not, with more awareness or not, with different traits and unique features, they will all find social interaction and social functioning challenging (Fletcher-Watson et al., 2013; White et al., 2015). Especially challenging is all forms of emotional and affectionate interpersonal communication. Therefore, in varying degrees, all people on the autism spectrum will find relating and relationships difficult.

Due to the wiring of their brain, all people who are not on the autism spectrum also have one thing in common. Whether introverted or extroverted, with different temperaments and different abilities and inabilities, they do not have the same structural differences in the regions of the brain that supports social interaction and social functioning as people with ASC do. They do not experience the same social challenges in the same way as people with ASC do. They do not find relating and relationships as challenging as people with ASC do.

These differences are hardwired. While there are degrees of difference, the brains of those with ASC are not at all like the brains of those who are NT. Lucy (NT) shared how attending a workshop had opened her eyes to an understanding of the specific brain differences:

She showed us the two brains, a picture of the two brains and all of us were so emotional because … we were blown away by the reality that 'Oh my God, that's their brain, that's my brain, they're distinctly different!'

These unique features to how the autistic brain work establishes distinctive behaviour. Noticeably different to neurotypical behaviour, the autistic brain is wired for more non-social activities. Accordingly, while all relationships undergo challenges, greater challenges will be experienced in relationships that include both people with ASC and people who are NT. The pairing of two distinctly different brains; a brain wired for solitary activities with a brain wired for social activities, will naturally trigger unconventional difficulties, and in turn, shape a very unusual type of relationship. However, due to the little-known features of autistic adults, this unusual type of relationship will be unknown to most.

In the two studies it was established that when people who have differently wired brains form a relationship together, a particular irregularity arises in their relationship. Due to characteristics of adults with autism, the same irregularities were observed in all neurodiverse relationships studied. Evolving into an unconventional interaction pattern that functioned in similar ways for each in these relationships, these irregularities triggered the formation of a specific dynamic. The neurodiverse dance – a dance in which the partners were truly out of step with each other.

Most NT participants spoke at length about being 'out of step' with their ASC partners and family members:

TRACY   *Often, my efforts at expressing warmth or affection were met with negative reactions, like I would come up behind James and touch him lovingly on his back or neck, and I would feel him stiffening up, as if I were a stranger! I didn't feel welcomed at all, so I stopped doing it … I get the impression that James does not understand what I am after. He doesn't know why I would not feel 'close' to him. He actually told me that he had no idea there was something amiss in our relationship for so long. I thought he was lying. He said: 'But we had three children together! But we bought a house together! You don't do such things with someone you are not close to!' It actually hurt me that he was in such an illusion for so long, we're talking something like 19 years here.*

SOPHIE   *One difficulty I have, is him not understanding those strange ways NTs communicate with each other. I will have to explain to him what certain actions mean or what an intent behind a conversation is. NTs are not literal like he sees the world. For example, I had to explain to him what mirroring is … in verbal affirmations such as, 'You are beautiful' or 'I love you'. I would end up telling him these verbal affirmations. He didn't understand this concept of mirroring. 'Why don't you just ask for what you want?' was his response. And here lies the differences of our two worlds of understanding.*

RUTH   *I would not describe my husband as warm or affectionate. I know he tries, but again, these things do NOT come naturally to him. He reports that he doesn't really 'feel warm' towards other people … Any declarations of love or affection are foreign and make him feel uncomfortable … Most of our conversations are exchanges of information. He has learned to ask me questions like 'How are you doing', 'How was your day', etc., but again, those things have not come naturally to him.*

RENEE   *I feel that my husband has no idea of me as a person. He struggles very much with understanding anything to do with me as a*

person, so he sees me as a physical person,
obviously, but really you scratch the surface,
and he doesn't know me at all.

LAURA   *I wish he paid me more attention, noticed me*
more, shared more of his inner life with me.
Wish he'd share activities with me. Sex would
be wonderful, but I accept that he can't/won't.
Often feel we just live two parallel lives. But
somehow there is a level of emotional intimacy,
paradoxically, and need on his part that makes
it more than a roommate situation.

On the other hand, participants with ASC described being 'out of step' in a different way:

SHARON   *I attempted to explain and expand using logical*
explanation. I have always been logical and
highly rational, which was one of the qualities
that attracted my partner, however this quality
gradually became a hindrance for emotional
connection for him.

WALLY   *Typically, I like being alone for a while and*
then I don't … then I miss being just around
in the house but … even when I'm in the
house I don't feel like we have to be conversing,
interacting whatever, all the time. I just want
to be in the same house. I read somewhere …
don't get the idea that all people with autism
just want to sit and rock in the corner. We
quite like to be social but we're really shit at
it.

Dancing with Difference

STELLA   *I mostly rely on sex to create an illusion of warmth and affection. We also discuss politics and have intellectual debates as a way to connect.*

Even though this same type of unique unconventional pattern appears to emerge in each neurodiverse relationship that includes both ASC and NT people, from the outside, these relationships do not look much different to regular relationships. As described in Book 1, most people on the autism spectrum become adept at camouflaging their autism in public (Mandy, 2019). Used as an adaptive mechanism to conceal differences and to achieve social acceptance, camouflaging autistic behaviour overcomes the appearance of 'different' when naturally not 'fitting in' to specific situations, especially social situations. Behind closed doors, however, is another story. In one's own home, the mask is discarded, the adaptive mechanisms are dispensed with, and the real person is revealed. Consequently, unseen and hidden to all but those inside the home, the characteristic autistic behaviours come to the fore. Only seen by those in the relationship, the unusualness of these relationships is strengthened by autistic behaviour that fluctuates between contexts inside the home as opposed to outside of the home.

Unless specifically trained in the nuances of autism's impact on relationships, formally or informally, whether in the role of counsellor, clinician, family member or friend, a lack of appropriate knowledge can lead to making judgements, offering advice, proposing treatments and therapies applicable to typical relationships, but downright harmful for neurodiverse relationships. The distinctive complications cannot be solved in typical ways. The differences in brain wiring means many of the challenges found in these relationships are not typical. While standard marital problems may have some bearing, focusing on them may obscure the specific complications that occur from hardwired differences.

Additionally, those in neurodiverse relationships often find the specific nuances of autism's influence difficult to convey to others. When reaching out for support, describing the details can be challenging. Often these challenges can further negative impressions, influence the inaccurate judgements of others and reinforce unhelpful therapies.

When attempting to explain the unconventionality of their relationships, most participants reported that they found it too complicated. Shirley (NT) shared why she had reservations about sharing:

Yeah, like if I try and explain the arguments that I've had with Jill to my NT colleagues who are social workers and in that field ha, ha. They find it very difficult. They just find it quite difficult to understand. Jill and I don't have the same arguments that other couples have, and a lot of NT people won't understand the whole Aspie way and the whole Aspie thinking and the sensory. Like if I try to tell my colleagues that I got into a fight with my partner because I touched her leg while she was eating her apple pie last night, like their ignorance on what sensory processing conditions are or autistic sensory issues will lead to them not believing ... so it's merely just their lack of understanding or knowledge on autism and if they hear all the things I have to do, or Jill kissing me before and after a shower, if they had an insight into our life here without the background and the years of knowing and learning about autism they would think we were quite strange. Yeah, they wouldn't understand.

Sophie (NT) also described how difficult it was to share her reality:

Unless someone has gone through a relationship like ours, there is no way for them to relate to this experience. There are both good and bad aspects to this type of pairing, but when we speak of things we talk to others about, we usually are referring to the negative aspects or problems. I find some friends incredibly judgemental of him, and us, so I retreat further away from them.

Likewise, Tracy (NT) had similar reservations:

I do not think that anyone can have just a bit of knowledge about AS and be able to believe or understand what we go through. A little bit of knowledge would, in my opinion, only lead to remarks such as: 'My husband is the same', or 'All men are like that'.

An anonymous survey respondent (NT) shared both her longing for a life that was beyond her reach but much too difficult to describe to others:

There's always going to be that longing for what will never be ... that longing for a life that only exists in fairy tales. What must it be like? To have a relationship with someone who 'gets you', to connect. I can only imagine. But I mustn't waste time wistfully wishing for something, as I know it's beyond him to 'get' me. I have an enviable life. He definitely loves me, about that I have no doubt, and he is so devoted, it's just something, something that's difficult to explain unless you've been there or are there.

Quinn (NT) revealed that the complexities were too hard to convey so she had decided not to tell her family:

Even when we actually have the diagnosis, I don't think we'll share it with our family ... My mum might understand a little bit. She seems to be a little bit more reasonable now she's getting older, I don't think his parents would accept it. Even when my husband shared my son's ADHD diagnosis with her, with the grandma, she just said 'I'm surprised that he has that because you two are normal'. That's what she said! ... I didn't agree with that comment ... I don't think his mum would ever accept it and she is very different lady, so I don't know, she might be on the spectrum too because she's just different, yeah.

Likewise, Wally (ASC) described the lack of belief he had experienced:

I find people do not believe the extent of the difficulties that I have personally in day-to-day activities and particularly because I function well at work.

A Dialogue Dance

While commonplace autistic behaviour kept hidden behind closed doors underpins the unconventional quality to these relationships, associated with these unseen aspects is the inherent social reciprocity difficulties of those on the spectrum (Kimura et al., 2020). As reported in Book 1, a lack of reciprocal conversation is a fundamental feature of neurodiverse relationships.

Reciprocal conversation is described by Dodd (2005) as the 'sharing of conversation, direction of an activity and resources' (p. 138). Keysar et al. (2008) describes it as working together on a common goal to create successful interaction by making adjustments until success is achieved. Whereas, Caruana et al. (2017) describes it as 'dynamic and reciprocal – your behaviour affects my behaviour, which affects your behaviour in return' (p. 115). Much like dancing together, the movement of one person influences and is influenced by the movement of another. Similarly, through the flowing exchange of words, nonverbal cues and appropriate responses, the comments of one person influences and is influenced by the comments of another. Achieved through multiple exchanges of asking questions, answering questions, building on each other's comments and listening carefully to know what to say next, all contributors equally share in this dialogue dance.

However, a defining characteristic of individuals with ASC is difficulty with giving and receiving reciprocal interaction (Sato et al., 2017). Asking questions, answering questions, building on another's comments and listening carefully are all vulnerabilities of autistic people, which adversely affects the ability to understand and respond to the thoughts and feelings of others. Consequently, the day-to-day giving and receiving of emotional and affectionate conversation that normally takes place in close relationships is unlikely to occur in most neurodiverse relationships.

Have We Gone Nuts?

Many NT participants described their partners and family member's difficulties in these areas and the impacts that it had on them:

ROSE *If I was asking for affection ... it makes him really panicked and overwhelmed and so I mean he's responding then but it's not the way that I would like a response. It turns into something very challenging, but it's just because he feels bad that he didn't understand or didn't notice and so it can be really hard to feel like you don't get something that other people get. So, that can turn into something pretty challenging for us because then he's panicky and I'm frustrated. But he's always responding it's not like he's not caring, it just doesn't always turn into the response that I would hope for.*

GEORGIA *The inability to just listen and comfort and just console. It's very cold, it's like living in a refrigerator ... I would be more willing to do that type of work if I felt I was getting at least some sort of reciprocity ... 'I appreciate this', anything. It's like a blank. It's like you need to do this for me because I've got Asperger's, and this is the way I am and tough. Yeah, can you just give something back ... Neurotypicals they do give back and that emotional connection is made, and it becomes a two-way thing and ... it's just so normal. Whereas I feel like with my husband I have to give and if he does anything for me and gives to me then I have to be so appreciative … I have to be like 'Oh my God! Thank you so much!'*

WANDA   *He doesn't respond … but it's like there's a problem going on and he doesn't realise that you're upset so unless you say something he's not going to respond at all so you might be more judgemental I suppose to try to provoke a conversation. Otherwise, it's like he doesn't realise and then even if you bring up something that is a problem in your relationship like I have at different times said things about myself, how I'm feeling, and I think from the way he reacts like after two or three days he seems to just react. His behaviour and the way he speaks will be just sort of normal for him as if we didn't even have that conversation … it seems to me that they listen to you expressing how miserable you're feeling and then it's sort of like that was just the change of the wind that day and then in a couple of days everything is back to normal. They forget that you actually were just trying to disclose to them how really hurt you've been by something.*

HOLLY   *I would wonder why he wasn't responding … so I mean I had a craving for more intimacy than I had, but it was never achieved.*

RUTH   *A willingness to talk through issues and listen to the other person is important in a relationship.*

Have We Gone Nuts?

An anonymous survey respondent (NT) stated:

Talk to any partner of someone with ASD and you find you have the same communication difficulties.

On the other hand, participants with ASC described their challenges with reciprocity:

TOM   *Ken has drawn me into deep conversations about feelings when he needed to resolve something. While the conversations were difficult for me, the result was good. I can recall times when I made an emotional response to something that angered me. This resulted in extended periods of discomfort. I see the value in trying to have a non-angry conversation about things that bother me. However, this type of conversation is still difficult for me, and I don't like it.*

TERRY   *She would like me to take the lead with conversation at times and ask questions rather than hang back … Only able to keep that up for a certain period of time before I need to back off.*

Whether clinician, counsellor, family member or friend, it is vital to be aware that the difficulties people with ASC have with giving and receiving reciprocal interaction will affect a relationship in unusual ways that may not be immediately evident. Sometimes, the camouflaging behaviour that many autistic people employ to conceal differences may hide the facts. Sometimes, a lack of disclosure for fear of disparagement may hide the facts.

Dancing Alone

While a lack of reciprocity contributes, in part, to the unconventional features of neurodiverse relationships, so too does the autistic need for solitude. Due to their different neurology, adults with ASC have a higher need to seek solitude to recover from and relieve the day-to-day tensions that often arise for them.

As described in Book 1, a need to avoid interaction is especially so when involved in the emotional elements of relating. Malcolm (ASC) described his need for solitude to escape the pressures of life:

> *The main thing is, if I go to my cupboard, the family knows it is nothing they have done. I have just gone to my cupboard. I just need that time out ... When I am in my cupboard sulking, having a Matilda moment, I am processing. Processing what happened. Why am I in here? How can I make it better? I don't want to do this again, and even when I am doing it, I am thinking 'Oh God, why am I treating Grace this way? Like, just ridiculous. I haven't talked to her for two days.' And I process that, and it takes time. Sometimes I just can't get out of that. It goes around and around in my head. But as time has gone on, I have learned, I can stop it, sometimes, almost instantly. I will have a Matilda, and an Aspie moment and then I'll, 'No there is a better way to do this.'*

Jim (ASC) described how he thought being apart from Dianne (NT) worked best for him:

Have We Gone Nuts?

When we are together … we are poles apart, okay, but when we are apart, I'm doing my thing, she is doing her thing, it is fine, no problems cause I'm not in her face.

With a preference for solitude or separate activities, autistic people tend to prioritise time engaged in the pursuit of special interests or time spent alone, above time spent with others. This need for solitude epitomises an autistic person's extremely single-minded and egocentric thinking. Coined in 1911 by Swiss psychiatrist Eugen Bleuler to describe withdrawal into one's inner world, the term 'autism' is 'derived from the Greek word "autos", meaning self, same, spontaneous; directed from within' (Uddin, 2011, p. 1). This egocentric focus of autism is not the same as being self-aware, which is defined as the ability to see yourself clearly and objectively through reflection and introspection. In basic terms, the difference between being self-aware and an egocentric focus relates to the effect that you have on others. Being self-aware is being able to notice and reflect on one's internal state, to appreciate that everyone else has feelings and thoughts of their own. You understand that you have a complex inner world; you understand that others have one too. On the other hand, an egocentric focus means that you are only considering matters from your own perspective. You prioritise what you want and how you feel, even if the needs of others are greater. When focused on yourself, it's hard to even notice what others want or need or how to interact with them in meaningful ways. Tracy (NT) described the absolute self-focus of her husband:

There have been times when he has suggested we go to the cinema, but it has been because he wanted to see a film. And often he'll just say, 'I'm off to the cinema', on his way out, and I won't be invited and won't know what he's going to see.

Dancing with Difference

Similarly, Laura (NT) shared how she was obligated to customise her relationship to accommodate her husband's desire to be on his own:

The compromise that I can't ask him for more companionship than he's willing to dole out. I live alone but without the full freedom to do anything I want whenever I want because of his needs, his schedule.

Ruth (NT) revealed that she took an active role in making certain she wasn't kept at a distance:

I feel that we would just mostly co-exist or be like roommates or people with the same children who just exchange information if I wouldn't take a very active role in the relationship.

On the other hand, Malcolm (ASC) shared how his egocentric focus affected him and his relationship with Grace (NT):

If Grace talks to me, if I take it personally, which evidently, I do, because it's about me, I don't say anything, but she wants to converse, but I don't have that ability. I can't. What you mean you want to talk about this? I'm right and you're wrong. You're doing your thing, there is nothing to talk about and then I run away ... When Grace is wanting to share information and I just hear noise, and like she might even just be saying a few words or a few sentences, but I just hear this 'Rah, rah, rah, rah'. And I will say 'Honey, honey, stop shouting', or like just to speak to me calmly. And she is. She is speaking to me very calmly.

45

Have We Gone Nuts?

For people with ASC, solitude and separate activities are coping mechanisms against emotional overload, burnout and depression. On the other hand, sometimes a time of solitude is not necessarily always a pleasant time, but a safe time. There may be a sense of loneliness, but it feels safer to be alone. Whether times of solitude are pleasant or unpleasant, the resulting separation from loved ones creates an unconventional relational pattern due to a need to avoid affection and connection in preference for separate activities. While this relational pattern is extremely unusual for close relationships, frequently, it becomes the norm in neurodiverse relationships.

The communication system that develops within this pattern, described in detail Book 1, underlies many unconventional aspects of neurodiverse relationships. However, since professionals, extended family or friends will rarely, if at all, observe these fundamental autistic behaviours or observe the resulting relational pattern, understanding of what takes place and its effect on each in the relationship will be negligible. Once understanding of these aspects occur, however, it will provide a framework to better support people in neurodiverse relationships.

Support Thoughts

According to imaging studies of the brain, the brains of people with autism show structural differences from those of non-autistic brains. These differences appear throughout the brain. Some parts of the brain may be larger or smaller, or there may be differences in the way that several parts of the brain are connected. Some studies have found increased activity in certain areas of the brain, such as the amygdala, which is involved in processing emotions such as fear and anxiety. Other studies have found decreased activity in other areas of the brain, such as the prefrontal cortex, which is involved in decision-making and social behaviour. It is important for awareness to grow that a paring of these differences in brain functioning create a very different type of relationship to the conventional, and that these types of relationships are common.

The next chapter describes some of the differences of autism that influences contrasts in the behaviours between each group of people in neurodiverse relationships. It details the noticeably distinctive relationships. It details the noticeably distinctive thinking of each group and what it means to a relationship when these differences converge. It illustrates how the distinctive mindsets of each create an unconventionality to these relationships that are not so much unique to the individuals in each relationship, but instead, is the driving force behind the formation of a unique type of relationship that was found, in these studies, to have commonalities across all neurodiverse relationships. It is important for family, friends and clinicians to be aware of these commonalities in order to address the general lack of belief about adult autism, be able to accept the accounts of those in neurodiverse relationships, and to know how to offer appropriately tailored support and comfort to people in these relationships.

3

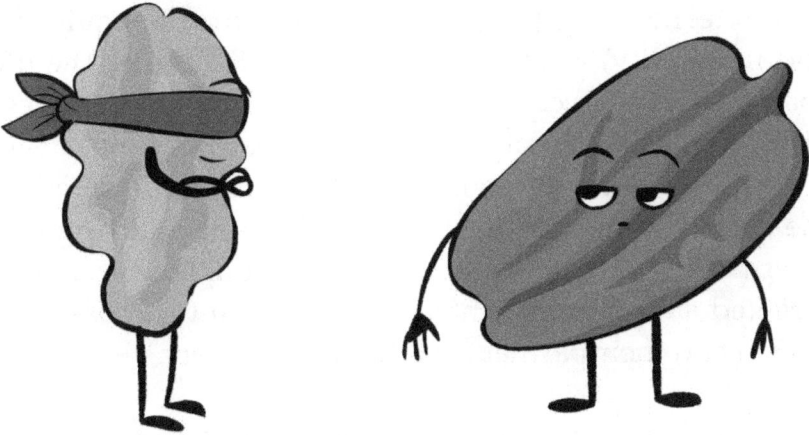

A Mysterious
Blindness

Have We Gone Nuts?

'Health is not a condition of matter, but of mind.'
Mary Baker Eddy

The Innermost Recesses

Difficulties with internalising (anxiety and low mood) and externalising (aggressive or outburst behaviours, and irritability) are very common in ASC across the life span (Ozsivadjian et al., 2021). Since it is known that these difficulties usually remain relatively stable over time but are often associated with poorer quality of life, understanding the cognitive mechanisms underlying internalising and externalising difficulties in ASC is essential for developing targeted supports and interventions, both for those with autism and their partners and family members.

Cognition refers to a range of mental processes related to the input and storage of information in the brain and how that information is then used to guide behaviour. Our cognitive abilities allow us to comprehend situations, discern what is required, and plan a course of action. We do this instinctively by reasoning, planning, solving problems, thinking abstractly, comprehending complex ideas and learning from experience (Karwowski & Kaufman, 2017).

However, due to a different neurology, people with ASC exhibit distinct patterns of cognition. The connectivity of the frontal lobes of the brain responsible for motor function, problem-solving, spontaneity, memory, language, initiation, judgement, impulse control and social and sexual behaviour operate in a unique way for those with autism (Catani et al., 2016; Lever & Geurts, 2016; Zeestraten et al., 2017). This difference is thought to lead to the distinctive way those with ASC think and perceive their world, while also influencing their understanding of the self, of others and their ability to relate and connect with others (Attwood, 2015).

It is vital to be aware that the cognitive differences between the two types of people are a fundamental characteristic of these types of neurodiverse relationships which is unlikely to be observed in any conventional close relationship. Even so, the resulting distinctive features may not be immediately evident. The camouflaging behaviour that many autistic people employ to conceal differences can hide related behaviours and the effects of those behaviours.

Three major cognitive theories (theory of mind, executive dysfunction and weak central coherence) have been hypothesised to underlie the core, defining symptoms of autism (Burnette et al., 2005; Joseph & Tager-Flusberg, 2004). While not the entire explanation, these theories appear to explain much about the cognitive differences that lead to the difficulties that people with ASC experience with social interaction, communicative capacity, and behavioural flexibility (the core triad of autism).

Seeing Blind

The term 'theory of mind' (ToM) is described as the ability to understand that other people have self-regulated, independent mental states, such as beliefs, desires, intentions, imagination and emotions and that these states are different to our own. This understanding helps us to interpret and predict other people's behaviour (Premack & Woodruff,

1978) or as Baron-Cohen (2008) describes it, 'the ability to put oneself into someone else's shoes, to imagine their thoughts and feelings' (p. 112). For that reason, a fully functioning ToM provides an implicit social 'know-how' that allows us to negotiate the mental domain (Hughes & Leekam, 2004). It allows us to connect, communicate and fully participate in the social world with others, and it makes possible that instinctive 'knowing' of how to react in any given situation.

People with ASC experience limitations with ToM (often referred to as mindblindness), which is one of the characteristic features of the ASCs, and is likened to being blind to the notion that there are other mindsets different to ones' own (Baron-Cohen, 1997; Baron-Cohen et al., 2001). This mindblindness undermines the ability to interact in socially normative ways (Brewer et al., 2017) and creates a fundamental difference in the way autistic individuals think and relate to others.

On the other hand, from an early age, neurotypical people acquire an understanding that other people have different mindsets to their own. They 'do not have to theorise that there are [other] minds as they can immediately experience other people's intentions and feelings within their affective, co-regulated interaction with them' (Williams , 2004, p. 704). It is a swift, frequently nonconscious process that aids in the processes of making sense of other peoples' behaviour (Williams, 2010). In other words, while not exactly a literal mind-reading ability, the act of participating in reciprocal emotional interaction is not unlike being able to 'read the mind of the other' through the reading of the entire verbal and non-verbal processes involved in an interaction.

A Mysterious Blindness

In these studies, the 'social know-how' differences between the two groups of participants created a fundamental contrast in how each dealt with the other. Winnie (NT) explained that her husband could only understand her emotional states if she made them obvious to him through very clear and observable behaviour:

> *He cannot express how he is feeling and similarly if I express how I am feeling his understanding is very limited … If I am very upset the only way that he will know is if I cry, then he will know, it's an obvious sign of distress, then he will quit and 'Oh she is upset'. If I am irritable or angry, its only if I speak sharply to him that he will have any idea that I might be irritable or angry, so his reading of me is very limited in an emotional scale so that makes our conversations quite stilted around emotions.*

Mary (ASC) described how her observations functioned to gauge another's demeaner:

> *I go a lot on sense, like how a person smells, how a person sits, how a person moves, more than anything on their face, or their tone of voice. I look at all factors of how a person is.*

Ryan's (NT) explanation of Rachelle's (ASC) inability to understand his needs displayed her mindblindness:

> *She doesn't understand illness, or my needs when ill. When she is ill, she needs nursing. She makes that clear and she is a bit of a sook about it sometimes, but other people, nuh, not much sympathy there.*

On the other hand, Rachelle showed some awareness of Ryan's discontentment with her when she noted:

He wants more constant connection throughout the day, he doesn't feel satisfied so he goes and does a lot of community things so he can connect with people because he's obviously not getting it from me.

Her mindblindness was evident in her answer to the question of how it affects her relationship:

I don't know, I can't tell. I think our relationship is fine.

Dianne (NT) explained that Jim's (ASC) inability to 'be aware' affected the way she responded to him:

If there were any response to show that 'Look I'm trying to be aware', and with all the knowledge and information that he has, I probably would react differently, but … to me, you are not making one slight effort to identify what could be done differently. Not that you have to be different, but to be more aware of who and what you are … there has been a real honest 'Yeah I'm Aspie, being Aspie means this is how I behave, this is what it does, I now realise', and for me it was a relief. He can't change it, but that doesn't mean he can't become more aware of it. Yeah, and that's what frustrates me, and I think, 'No there are people out there that are Asperger's that at least make a bit more of an effort.' Yeah, so, I still don't think that there is total self-acceptance.

Then she added:

A Mysterious Blindness

I really believe that there is things outside of being Aspie with Jim ... like his whole upbringing, that have also impacted on the fact that he just won't see – well he understands that he is Aspie, but he won't see his behaviours. I think that's outside of Aspie, we all get influenced by our backgrounds and where we have come from, and if you are Aspie that only probably makes it more difficult.

Whereas Jim's explanations revealed his mindblindness:

I don't necessarily know what I do wrong, so there is a lot of issues there that you think, 'What can I do better?' What do you mean better? Do what better? I have been to courses where, I just did a course recently at Minds and Hearts ... for guys who were suffering from Asperger's, and we had exercises to do and I'm thinking, 'Mate I'm wasting my bloody time ... because I wouldn't be able to get my explanation out quick enough or out enough so that she would understand.' Ah, it would have been a fruitless exercise ... All these other guys, they were talking to their wives, and am thinking 'Yes, but none of those people have got my wife and she's pretty bitter about the whole thing, because she just feels that I'm not trying.' But the point is, 'What are you supposed to be trying at?' ... We've been there for psychological help and all that sort of stuff, but again if you don't know what's broken, how do you fix it? That's why I'm such a good handyman, because I can actually see it and I can fix it ... Something tangible I can fix. Something psychological or emotional, nah, nah sorry, it's not in my spectrum.

Likewise, rather than attempt to gain some understanding of what was needed to repair a personal problem, Tom (ASC) said that he just waited for it to be over:

Have We Gone Nuts?

Sometimes if he seems distant, I wait for him to be not distant.

Making his mindblindness obvious, he added:

Sometimes I notice him looking at me so I look at him and smile, but I think he might be trying to send a non-verbal message that I don't understand.

Wally's (ASC) conversation revealed how mindblindness obstructed an ability to overcome his circumstances:

My wife was probably resisting being my carer so the relationship kind of broke down a bit there and particularly the physical intimacy side of that pretty much disappeared. So we talk but I'm probably not very good at recognising what or how to offer emotional support there and because the physical side of our relationship has largely disappeared that mode of communication is no longer available and I don't know how you get it back.

However, Terry (ASC) saw the humour in it:

Ha, ha, ha. It's the unknown, unknown.

Although the difficulties that autistic people have with recognising mental states in others is well-known, mounting evidence suggests that particular difficulties with an awareness of the 'psychological self', or 'theory of own mind' is an equal problem (Williams, 2010). Several studies have found that autistic individuals experience diminished and/or atypical features of self-awareness due to a delay in the development of self-insight. For example, Lind and Bowler (2009) confirmed that people with ASC have difficulty identifying and reflecting on their own mental states, as well as their own emotions. Dritschel et al. (2010) established that autistic adolescents often judge others as knowing as much about their own internal feelings (such as sadness, tiredness, etc.) as themselves, rather like young children do. However, in the general population, as people mature, they regard themselves as the only ones to have this type of knowledge. Huggins et al. (2021) verified that autistic adults had poorer emotional self-awareness compared to neurotypical peers, and Williams et al. (2018) concluded that, although neurotypical people found it easier to perceive and remember information that relates to themselves, people with autism showed features of self-awareness only when involved in non-emotional tasks.

Williams' (2010) study offered some explanations. Since awareness of mental states in both self and others develop in parallel, both can be similarly affected for autistic people. Additionally, Williams found that in some circumstances, the self-awareness of those with ASC of their own mental states was found to be even more affected than their awareness of mental states in others. By regularly observing others' actions, it can provide an opportunity to learn 'behaviour rules', regarding the behaviour of others. However, one's own behaviour is rarely observed so opportunities to learn self-behaviour rules are less frequent (Williams, 2010). Given that a self-concept guides and controls behaviour (Markus & Wurf, 1987), without both self-awareness and other awareness, interpersonal interaction can become extremely challenging.

Mary (ASC) confirmed that was the case for her. She reflected on trying to decipher her inner world:

Have We Gone Nuts?

There are a few other things that people say, and I would just look at them and go 'I've got no clue what you are talking about.' ... some things in my own process I am generally quite enlightened, in other people's processes I have no idea. In saying that, I still don't really understand my own emotions. I really don't understand. I only know that they exist, and they must exist for a reason, because emotions are an important tool to alert us to psychological distress or psychological workings, so they exist for a reason, so therefore, I must pay attention to them. Because it is part of my survival as a human being, but that's as far as I get, so I kind of understand the reason why I have them biologically speaking, because it's part of being human, but when I have them, I go, 'What am I feeling? I am feeling something really strong, but I've got no idea what it is.' And it's usually because my guts are all, or I've got a headache or I've got that pressure, or my teeth hurt. I get this physiological symptom, and I think 'Oh, I must be feeling something. What am I feeling? Well, it must be strong because these sensations are strong, therefore it is sending me a message. Why am I getting the message? Oh my God. Shit. Shit' So yeah, I am enlightened in the process, but am not enlightened. I've got terrible emotional intelligence. If I could live without emotion, I would be quite happy.

Then she added:

I don't know if that makes it easy. I think it makes it both easier and harder for both groups. Because some people are very good at shoving it under the carpet. The thing is ... once I know what it is, I will confront it head on. I will go 'Right. Okay then.' Once I understand what's going on. And then I am not afraid of it anymore. I just go 'Oh yeah, I can see why I would feel that way. That's pretty shit. Alright then.'

A Mysterious Blindness

And now I either stay away from it, whatever is making me feel that way, whether it's a person, place or thing, because I figure if that person, place or thing is going to make me feel that way, then they are not worth having. So nowadays, to me that's logic.

Brought to a Standstill

Executive dysfunction is another major cognitive theory that has been hypothesised to underlie the core, defining characteristics of autism. Executive function is an umbrella term that refers to a set of cognitive processes essential to goal-oriented behaviour, such as planning, organisation, decision-making, problem-solving and logical analysis that controls other lower-level cognitive processes such as motor activity, sensation, perception, attention or memory (Braden et al., 2017; Johnston et al., 2019). Like theory of mind, executive function is associated with the integrity of the frontal lobe (Brady et al., 2017).

Executive function is required to adapt to novel or complex situations, adjust to the many multidimensional social rules, manage the changing nature and needs of relationships, and the know-how to make required amendments when needed (Braden et al., 2017; Happé et al., 2006; Johnston et al., 2019). In other words, executive function is 'the dimension of human behaviour that deals with "how" behaviour is expressed' and makes independent and productive behaviour possible (Jurado & Rosselli, 2007, p. 213).

When experiencing difficulties with executive functioning, it can adversely affect independent functioning. Consequently, people can struggle to get anything done, which can lead to a lack of motivation to put effort into things that appear too hard or neglect the activities that are required for independent success. However, as adults, we are expected to be able to do things independently and function on our own. We need to be capable of completing our daily tasks on time, proficiently shift between different tasks in a timely manner, organise our day at work and at home and regulate our behaviour appropriately through all the circumstances that life brings.

For those with ASC, executive dysfunction creates difficulties with engaging in independent and purposeful behaviour (Jurado & Rosselli, 2007). It also creates difficulties with effective problem-solving abilities (Zelazo et al., 2003), complications with attention, working memory and fluency (Braden et al., 2017) and problems with adaptive behaviour and cognitive flexibility (Granader et al., 2014; Pugliese et al., 2016).

Interviews revealed the consequences of cognitive differences between the groups of participants. Georgia (NT) shared her husband's description of his cognitive processes:

When we have conversations, he said, 'You can move so fast and switch so quickly, I cannot keep up, the speed which you get from things and make connections … I'm left lagging behind. By the time I've processed one thing that you've said and felt the emotion that's connected with that one thing that you've said, you've already moved on to the next thing.' Because that's the way we are. It's so natural. There is no thought for us. It's just instinctual. It just comes, whereas he has to hear it, think it, process it, then feel it, then process it, think it and then respond, and that sometimes when you're talking to them, they just go quiet. You ask them and you're like 'respond', and they don't respond, and I'm thinking that must be what they're doing. They're thinking and they're processing and they're trying to understand what it is you said, and that was one thing that I learnt to do that when I am talking, because … I talk a lot and I talk really quickly, is to try and slow down and when I ask him something don't expect an answer straight away just give him the time to process and sometimes you have to actually prod and give him clues.

Whereas Wanda (NT) revealed how Wally (ASC) did not think ahead or plan for the changing nature and needs of the family:

He actually told me he was going to Melbourne; he's got this week and then in two more weeks he's going away for another week. I said, 'Oh lucky I hadn't applied for, or hadn't got any graduate position yet because somebody has to be here for my daughter', and he goes 'Well you'd be still there.' I was like 'Yeah, but if I'm nursing, I could be on night shifts or evening shifts or anything. We have to plan ahead if you're going to be going away … somebody needs to be here.' He didn't seem to get it at all. It was really weird.

Ruth (NT) illustrated some of the repercussions of their executive functioning differences:

We have the same conversations over and over, and I think he understands what I am saying and where I am coming from. We agree to take some course of action on a particular issue, and then it's like he 'forgets' and just goes and does it the way he is comfortable with or the way he has 'always done it', which often looks selfish to me, like he isn't taking my thoughts and feelings into consideration.

Quinn (NT) described her husband's lack of goal-oriented behaviour:

He complains a lot about his job. It's very stressful. It's a lot of work so I say, 'Well are you going to look into something else ... so I would find programs for him, and he'll be like, 'Yes, I'm going to go and do a master degree', and then eight months go by and he never does anything and then I bring it up again and he might say he's going to do it and then he never does it so it's kind of like that and then that's why it's never resolved ... like if I want closet shelves, he might tell me, 'Let's go to the store'. We'll look at them and he comes back and says, 'I'm going to measure everything and you're going to get your closet.' And a year goes by, two years and I never get the closet.

Rae (NT) shared how she dealt with a lack of goal-oriented behaviour:

It's hard to get him to make a decision, but I sort of give him ultimatums now, you know, 'I want this done, I want some action and I want it done by the end of the week.'

Katy (NT) revealed that Ronald (ASC) did not have the executive functioning to maintain his appearance without her support:

He needs to ask me whether he needs a shave or whether he needs any other clothes on or he still seems to rely on me for keeping himself physically looking okay. So, he's a bit eccentric in that way and can look extremely ... scruffy.

A Mysterious Blindness

Renee (NT) explained that her remedy to the situation was to organise everything herself:

If I wanted to go away, I would have to organise it myself, and put everything in place, and tell him about it later, which is basically what I did. He really didn't have to do anything, and I explained it to him in a way that was just like 'Well this is what's going to happen and here's what you need to do', which in most relationships that is not how you do things, but he was just absolutely okay with that.

Similarly, Dianne (NT) described how she was the one who needed to take action:

Things don't get done, and that drives me nuts ... I do it myself or just lose it and go, 'For God's sake how long do I have to wait to get this done?' And then I get all the excuses as to why and I just go, 'Well bloody just go and do it', and often that is a motivation and he will go and do it, or he will be pigheaded and just leave it for another couple of days ... It is something that I guess has come up at meetings. A lot of the ladies say that they give instructions about various things, and I initially thought, 'Oh no.' But I do, if things need to be done, I write a list. You know, of tasks to be done [be]cause they are not good planners ... Jim has one day a week off now, and if I don't put a list down to go, these things need to be done, he would just sort of kind of fart around for the day.

When asked how she felt about it, she added:

Well again, you are the fixer, you are the direction given ... you're the one who has to take charge again, and feel like a

mother, or a carer, or a do this, do that, like with your kids
… So, it is just frustrating. You are taking charge again. You
are having to make decisions again … having to take on the
burden again … it's that sharing thing that doesn't happen.
It is not, 'Let's do this together', 'What do you think', 'cause
they don't have an opinion. It is like, 'Well I don't know so
you tell me.' Yeah, it's just annoying.

An anonymous survey respondent (NT) shared the
difficulties that her husband's executive dysfunction made
for her life:

My husband has a complete lack of executive functioning
skills that is getting worse as he gets older and makes my
life a cul-de-sac. He cannot initiate or prioritise tasks, plan
ahead for even the next hour, gets the 'wrong end of the
stick' in most situations and needs the simplest of tasks
and requests to do things explained in detail. He cannot
remember conversations or events, and often just makes
things up from what he has seen on TV or on a billboard.
We have no history in the sense that I cannot reminisce
about anything with him. He needs context explained to him
otherwise he brings up inappropriate things with the wrong
people. He laughs in movies when nobody else is. All this
and we have our own business employing 10 staff and if I
am not 'supervising' every day, chaos and confusion can
ensue. If I am not there, he does not understand which are
the important things he needs to communicate to me, and
which are the things that can be left. He raises inappropriate
and irrelevant issues in staff meetings despite the agenda I
painstakingly create and give him each week. I waste hours
following up on unpaid bills, forgotten wages, reorganising
patients because he has not communicated he will be away,

and tasks he said he would do but has not even commenced. Our relationship would improve if he just got a carer and a personal assistant, and I left.

Executive functioning difficulties is considered to include cognitive inflexibility. Cognitive inflexibility is a facet of executive dysfunction which can explain some of the behavioural inflexibility in autism. It refers to the tendency to focus on one's own thoughts, beliefs or activity/behaviours often to the exclusion of most others, which can also be called 'mono-tropism' (Ozsivadjian et al., 2021). Cognitive inflexibility limits flexible problem-solving, inhibition of the current thought and smooth transition from one thought/ behaviour to another (Ozsivadjian et al., 2021).

Malcolm (ASC) shared how he put tasks and responsibilities into systems that he wanted all in his household to follow:

I want to give instructions to make things better ... I like systems. If I give direction, just do it. It's like a system ... I get all the work out of the way before I go and read my book, or before I eat, I will make sure all my jobs are done so when I eat, everything is calm, and all the dishes are put away. 'Well why don't you put all the dishes away?' It doesn't make sense. Course it makes it easier, otherwise you've got to do it after the meal ... If it is a job ... like cleaning the toilets, I will just do it because it is part of a system. It has to be done. Vacuuming, or housecleaning, or garden maintenance.

However, he recognised that it didn't always work that way:

Have We Gone Nuts?

So, and if people don't do that, I mean I am learning too, to deal with that ... I realise that people do things differently.

Grace (NT) agreed with Malcolm's descriptions and explained the reasons behind it:

So, you know, if there's chores to do, he will get them all done, and then he will go and retreat, and have something to eat, or read his book, or play a game, or whatever it is and sometimes that will be 10 o'clock at night before he is finished doing the things that he doesn't want to do, but has to do. So, he is very diligent. I mean, I would love to say 10 out of 10, but I am sure he would probably say he is not that perfect. So, I reckon nine, oh so I suppose there are other things apart from chores, so I suppose eight ... there are things like social stuff. I will probably say eight, if something is left undone, he will get stressed. So, it is actually more stress for him to not complete than to complete, for him. So even if ... it took two or three weeks, that is irrelevant to him. It is on his list; it has to be crossed off. That's how he is ... He manages it so systematically ... he has a system for everything ... if something freaks him out, as long as you give him cupboard time to digest it, he is brilliant. He just goes in there, does it, sorts it, and comes out.

Like Malcolm, Mary (ASC) also described how she was often compelled to complete tasks without delay:

My whole life is about fulfilling tasks, fulfilling roles, being a person that needed to appear a certain way. Whereas now I actually make a concerted effort to cognitively negate. So, when I instinctively go to do something, I am mindful about it. I go 'Okay, do I really need to do this right now, or can wait a few hours, a couple of days?'

Attention to Detail

A third major cognitive theory also hypothesised to underlie the core, defining symptoms of autism is weak central coherence. Central coherence is defined as being able to understand the meaning and/or point of view. It is the ability to determine meaning from a collection of details; to draw information from different sources, experiences and representations, both internal and external, and to put them together to make sense of circumstances and to formulate meaning from them (Booth et al., 2003; Happé & Frith, 2006). In other words, the difference between seeing a forest when looking at a large group of trees, or only seeing an assortment of individual trees.

Weak central coherence is a specific perceptual-cognitive style that limits the abilities of those with ASC to understand context or be able to comprehend configural information (that is, the big picture). Rather, they show a propensity to focus mainly on details (Attwood, 2007; Lovett, 2005). This cognitive style can leave individuals vulnerable to the misinterpretation of situations and communications, as a tendency to focus on details limits the ability to understand context or to comprehend the bigger picture (Booth et al., 2003; Loth et al., 2010).

While focusing on details can be a strength in certain circumstances, without an ability to give attention to the bigger picture, when required, adults with ASC will not be able to recognise the relevance of different types of knowledge or information within a particular situation, to appreciate what is more important over what is less important. A higher level understanding will, therefore, not be gained in order to grasp what decisions need to be made, or the action to take, relevant to that situation (Lovett, 2005). Wally (ASC) said that was the case for him:

> *I think I've done the right thing, said the right thing but I can't understand, I can't clearly understand the effect.*

Sophie (NT) described the impact of her partner's lack of 'big picture' thinking on the both of them:

> *Some concepts or conversations I can come back to at a later time and discuss them when he is in a better emotional place. Other times I just need accept he won't understand … The simplest thing he could do to help better understand me is to ask questions for clarification versus assume a meaning in a communication. He often will apply a meaning to something that is far from what was intended based on his filter of how he interprets things … I will attempt to change the way the conversation is phrased, or I will use a different approach. Often, I will use a third-party type example. He sometimes does not understand the direct effect of his actions on others, but if I phrase the action or conversation where he is the recipient of the offensive behaviour, a clarity comes over him. He usually will apologise and be sad after knowing the hurt he caused intentionally or unintentionally.*

Similarly, Rose (NT) spoke about the resulting impact on each other of inabilities to comprehend meanings:

> *Maybe like 30% of what I'm trying to convey, and I maybe understand 30% of what he's trying to convey ha, ha … but it's better than zero. We eventually, if something happens that we have a really big miscommunication and we're really*

frustrated, usually we separate and then like 45 minutes later we'll come back and talk about it … for us it's more about communication. We have different types of challenges, but they end up getting handled the same way.

Thinking Absolutely

A relatively new cognitive theory has been gaining ground. An aspect of the central coherence hypothesis, its specific focus is on perception of context. Vermeulen (2015) points out that contextual sensitivity is a part of the central coherence hypothesis 'that has been largely overlooked in both literature and scientific research, namely, the ability to use context in sense making' (p. 182). He coined the term 'context blind' to describe this difficulty. Vermeulen (2015) proposes that people with autism lack contextual sensitivity which plays a vital role in a number of cognitive processes, such as: seeing relevance and guiding attention; face processing; disambiguation of meaning in language and communication; understanding human behaviour and actions; and, flexibility in problem-solving and generalisation of knowledge and skills (Vermeulen, 2015; Westby, 2017). Being context blind means that people with ASC give meaning in an absolute, rather than in a contextually sensitive manner, however, the meaning of almost every situation in life is context dependent (Vermeulen, 2012, 2015).

Vermeulen (2012, 2015) also puts forward the idea that since there are no absolute meanings in our world; everything that we do, think and say is context dependent; therefore, people with autism are absolute thinkers in a relative world. However, contextual sensitivity fosters the ability to navigate a world full of ambiguity. If people with ASC do not have contextual sensitivity to draw upon, they become blind to the use of context in the creation of meaning. Vermeulen (2012) suggests that others should clarify the context of each situation for them so that people with autism can find their way less blindly in a word full of relative meanings; that contextual clarification is the core of 'autism friendliness' (p. 378). However, providing contextual clarification within interactions, while helpful, could become a factor in the development of other problems, such as dependency on others to prompt, guide, instruct and explain social nuances. Explained in Book 1, an ongoing requirement to instruct, explain or in this case, clarify context, may result in overburdening others which can develop into a parental caretaker role. Kay's (NT) description illustrated the extent of assistance required to provide contextual clarification:

> *'Did you understand what I was feeling or what I meant before? Or how that went?' So it is constantly going back and reminding and reminding this is what happened. This is how I felt. This is what I need. Again. And can we move forward and have an agreed way forward? And consistently going back to that. Going back to that until it is almost like a habit.*

Crucial to being successful in relationships is having a **fully functioning ToM** to provide the social 'know-how' to make sense of other peoples' behaviour, **executive functioning** to adapt to and manage the changing nature and needs of relationships, **central coherence** to understand meanings and/or point of view and **contextual sensitivity** to understand that most situations in life are context dependent. Equally, our experiences with the social world, both internally and externally, allows us to function well socially and to accomplish typical behaviour in social situations (Arioli et al., 2018; Schaller & Rauh, 2017).

Accordingly, our social cognition is at the basis of all communicative and otherwise interpersonal relationships (Baez & Ibanez, 2014). Casanova (2019) points out, however, that anatomical abnormalities in the cerebral cortex of the autistic brain contributes to their poor cognitive and social functioning. The cerebral cortex enables us to process sensory information, engage in complex thought and abstract reasoning, and produce and understand language. Malcolm (ASC) shared the mental workout his thinking processes required him to go through to interact with others:

See when I meet someone, I examined their body, posture, the way their hands move, how their face is moving. I am wondering when they say something, what are you actually saying? What do you mean by that? How are you saying it? Why are you saying that? How do you want me to respond? Am I standing the right way? What do I need to do? Do I need to smile now? Do I have to say something back to you? Do I just stare at you? You know, all that kind of stuff. That's what's going through my head every time I talk to someone ... Oh, mate. Hahaha. Some days, I will tell you, just taking the kids to school. You know, every morning, I have to think. I will see someone in the distance. Well first of all, I will prepare myself in the head. I have got to do the school run. I might see this person. I might see this person. I've got to see the teacher. What have I got to say to the teacher? How do I act with the teacher? What do I do with the children? Do I walk them in this way? How do I act? What do I have to say to them? How do I look after them

71

emotionally? Does [my son] need a cuddle this morning? I
haven't given him a cuddle, so I need to cuddle him. He is
a human, so he needs me.

Therefore, when compromised in these domains, the social
cognition inabilities of those with ASC leads to difficulties
understanding what to say to others and how to respond to
them. These inabilities underpins problems with aspects such
as thinking about other people's thoughts and intentions to
understand and predict others' behaviour, social inattention,
difficulties with empathising with others and a lack of
motivation to be social (Arioli et al., 2018). Malcolm (ASC)
also described his fluctuating social motivation:

If it is socially, like going for a cup of tea with Grace the
other night, I know it's important. We have an agreement
with each other that if she says 'It's important. I need you
to be there', I will. I would deal with it and do it. But if I
have a choice, I won't, in that kind of situation. So, I think
the motivation changes depending on how planet Malcolm
sees it, of course.

However, an interesting factor was found in the study
conducted by Baez and Ibanez (2014). In their study,
participants with ASC functioned well socially when explicit
social information was presented or when the situation
could be navigated with abstract rules (Baez & Ibanez, 2014).
Similarly, in my studies it was found that some adults with
ASC were able to learn how to navigate some of the nuances
of social interaction when provided concentrated assistance
from NT partners or family members. Sophie (NT) described
some of her direct and to the point communication techniques:

A Mysterious Blindness

I will clearly tell him things like, 'I need you to hold me for a bit', 'I am going to kiss you now', 'Will you please say encouraging or loving things to me', etc. I have to be acutely aware of my own needs and then communicate them to him in a very straightforward manner, so he knows what he needs to do ... but usually [he] applies his own needs first – typical Asperger's. He does notice my physical affections and when I am direct in my verbal communication with him. I have taken numerous upper-level communication courses to help understand more about communication and how to apply things to our relationship in order to improve things.

Similarly, an anonymous survey respondent (NT) described some of the explicit communication techniques and guidelines used to facilitate communication:

Have to learn skills other than the usual social skills in order to have successful communication with an Aspie. For example, have to think in advance about how to frame requests in terms of what he would get out of it. Have to think prior to raising issues about how to say things in a way that he will receive them. Have to be more rational and not emotive at all. As soon as any emotion is involved, he shuts down, so spontaneous discussions don't happen.

Through the lens of cognitive theories, it is evident that the social cognitive and social functioning contrasts between ASC and NT people plays a part in triggering the unconventional quality seen in these relationships. Consequently, it is essential to understand that differences between ASC and NT people are not merely behavioural or relational. The distinctive contrasts between these two types of people are due to very definite brain differences. When a relationship forms between them, these contrasts need to be understood in the context of a pairing of dissimilar brains, as well as the usual considerations of personality and individual differences of each, to be able to offer appropriate services and support.

Inwardly Blind

Although cognitive theories account for some of the differences between ASC and NT people, they are not the whole story. As Lombardo and Baron-Cohen (2011) explain, 'people do not exist in a vacuum. We are "selves" embedded in a rich social world full of other "selves"' (p. 131). Our environment, interactions and relationships with others, background, culture and life experiences, similarly have bearing on shaping each 'self'.

Typically, a person's concept of self consists of all the characteristic attributes, conscious and unconscious, mental and physical aspects of that person which involves self-esteem, self-worth, self-image and identity. Therefore, a sense of self is a combination of the way we see ourselves, how we feel about ourselves, together with our experiences and environments. Our perception of ourselves is important because it affects our motivations, attitudes and behaviours.

According to Parise et al. (2019) a clearly defined self-concept is not only positively associated with one's wellbeing, but also with one's relational wellbeing. A person who is aware of their strengths and weaknesses, the nature of their personalities, and where they stand on important attitudes and values is more likely to be satisfied with themselves and within their relationships. Your self-concept impacts the questions you typically ask yourself each day, how you interact with people and how you think about yourself, others and your circumstances. Therefore, your self-concept basically determines what you will or will not do and what you will or will not say at any given moment in time.

Studies of the self in autism have found that from an early age, people with ASC exhibit atypical interpretations of themselves (Burrows et al., 2017). Research data on self-recognition reveals that autistic children's responses to their mirror images are qualitatively different from those of typical children (Lyons & Fitzgerald, 2013). Measured by a self-recognition test, children with ASC show little interest in their own mirror images and have been described as relatively 'face inexperienced' leading to differences in the development of self-awareness (Lyons & Fitzgerald, 2013). Coutelle et al. (2020) found that the perception of themselves can be inaccurate, attributable to 'a lower clarity of self-concept and a lower social function of autobiographical memory' (or memory of the self) (p. 3874). Huang et al. (2017) found that there are variations in self-awareness for individuals with ASC at most levels that include the following:

- They do not know what they do not know, so it is hard for them to judge when and how to know more
- They have difficulty telling the differences between their own or others' preferences and emotions in social situations
- They have difficulty relating their own behaviours to environmental and social contexts/situations, and to others' actions
- They have difficulty understanding self and others' thoughts and feelings.

Have We Gone Nuts?

Barry (ASC) evaluated how his lack of self-understanding led to difficulties figuring out the specifics of problems:

> *I wouldn't be able to pinpoint what, if someone said, 'Okay now what's the problem?' You know, managed to find a counsellor say, and then I don't know how to answer that. I would go 'Uh, ah, yeah, good question. Ah I don't know.' A lot of the time, you can't put your finger on what you think is wrong.*

Quinn (NT) described how her partner's lack of self-understanding led to an inability to have a conversation with him:

> *Our conversations, usually it just goes one way. I talk, and he listens. If I ask anything he takes forever to answer. Most times he tells me he doesn't know, like if I ask, 'Why did you do this?' He'll just say he doesn't know, and I always thought he was just saying that, but after talking to him again this week it really does seem like he just doesn't have a clue. Sometimes he makes decisions, and he doesn't think through, so I think truly that's all he can answer, that he doesn't know because truly he doesn't know. So, he doesn't really give me anything back for me to work with, it's really not a conversation, it's just me talking and him responding if he has to but most times he won't even respond.*

One's concept of self is an important aspect in the development of our social and cognitive functioning. It is at the basis of our abilities to read the mental states of others, form a healthy self-other differentiation in relationships and manage the self in a way that is socially acceptable. It is not only a vital aspect to managing oneself, but also in the maintenance of effective relationships.

A Mysterious Blindness

Due to their different neurology, Nguyen et al. (2020) found that 'autistic adults perceive themselves as having a low sense of power in their relationships and have negative global perceptions of their self-worth. However, those able to find positive meaning or benefits associated with autism are likely to have more positive global self-perceptions' (p. 1). When Max (ASC) was asked how he was able to come to a place of acceptance and to receive Mia's (NT) instruction, he replied:

> I think that depends largely on the type of person you are, whether you are open to learning new things or not and that applies to neurotypicals as well as people on the autistic spectrum. If you don't have the humility to respond to your external suggestions you don't improve either way. Now in my case I was actually very, very conscious of the fact that I was doing something wrong from a very early age. I remember being in year 6, year 7 thinking to myself I wish someone would tell me what I'm doing wrong and always conscious of not being able to socialise properly and so I was always open to the idea that someone would help me, so that's where I was coming from, but I guess if you don't have that desire to learn or that ... willingness to learn then that itself would be an impediment to learning you know.

However, research has also found that many people with ASC who have higher IQ may be aware of their social insufficiencies but may be unable to address them appropriately. Wally (ASC) described how he was trying to come to terms with the knowledge of his difficulties and to help others in the process:

Have We Gone Nuts?

I've got a PhD; I've got a Doctorate ... I think I've done the right thing, said the right thing but ... I can't clearly understand the effect ... and in terms of what I put on the survey, I don't really know what I need. I don't know how much I need ... If somebody asked me to talk to Faculty about ASD students or the experience, I never say no and that's why I did the PhD in the first place you know, partly to understand myself but partly to be part of that contribution.

The outcomes of atypical representations of 'self' may not be immediately evident to external others since the camouflaging behaviour that many autistic people employ to conceal differences can hide related conduct and its effects. However, it is vital to be aware that due to the two different neurology's between the two types of people in neurodiverse relationships, there is a pairing of very different concepts of 'self'. These differences will affect the behaviour of each in a way that is unlikely to be observed in any conventional close relationship. Wally (ASC) also described the difference between the perceptions held within, as opposed to outside, his relationship:

I've definitely been through times where I wish I didn't know. I've lived in blissful ignorance for 38 years just thinking that other people were the problem, and she just kind of put up with it. I believe that I've changed ... we've talked about, 'Okay so now I'm an Aspie husband and now I'm Aspie Wally' and she says, 'No. You're just Wally, you know. You haven't actually changed that much', but I'm so much more aware of who I am and what I say, if not actually in the moment, then soon afterwards. I make a lot of mistakes in social and relationships. I manage perfectly fine at work and I'm in a fairly senior position so I can afford to, people forgive me because I'm the

*boss and I've talked about that with staff ... that you know I
can get away with being eccentric or a little bit rude sometimes
because I'm the boss you know and I usually figure it out and
come around afterwards and say, 'Oh yeah, sorry that didn't
quite work out' you know and I'm very open about being on
the spectrum and in my organisation roughly 30% of our
students claim a disability and that's disclosed and a pretty
high percentage of those would be ASD ... the environment
that I work in has very high numbers of students with ASD
and staff as well. Some of them who know about it, some of
them who don't, quite a few who know about it now, that
didn't know about it before they met me. There have been
several staff members who have actually had diagnoses since
they've known me out of the 260-odd faculty.*

Captivated by Specialties

Lyons and Fitzgerald (2013) suggest that while there is
substantial evidence to suggest that an atypical sense of self
in autism contributes to their differences in the social and
communication domains, it might also contribute to their
talents and special skills. In other words, while problematic
for the social areas of life, this diminished self-awareness in
autism might aid in the development of special gifts (Lyons
& Fitzgerald, 2013). Rose (NT) described the advantages:

*My brother's special interest is computers and he's been taking
them apart and putting them together and programming
computers since he was five, and he's really good at it ...
[My husband is] ... naturally inclined towards being good
at music, he doesn't think he's super great at it but he is,
and he can play 15 instruments.*

Have We Gone Nuts?

Ronda (NT) described both advantages and disadvantages:

The tragic day that I lost him was the day he got his first computer. He's just become addicted to his computer. That's his life. That's his universe now, but before we had computers … we would spend our evenings listening to music together and talking about music we would listen to. We would buy records together at the record store and then be really excited to go home and listen to them together. We would be playing music together. When one of us discovered some new music, we would share it with the other person and have them listen to it and we would comment and discuss it and have dinner together. We did things together, we played music together, we were in a music group together and we would sit around and compose songs together … We still had a social life, mainly because I had a group, was a professional musician so I had a lot of friends through the music and the day he got his first computer I lost him. That's when I really lost him. He just changed worlds and went into his computer world and never came out.

Terry (ASC) also described this intense focus and how it shut everything else out:

I've realised it only probably in the last couple of years that if I'm in the zone or flow with something I'm actually doing that's visual and tactile my hearing shuts down and Kim will be saying things … and I just haven't heard it. It's not so bad the other way around if I'm listening intently to some music, I tend to miss things in my visual field. I don't think it's anywhere near as much as once the visual system takes over, that does cause a lot of communication problems so when Kim is trying to talk to me about something I've zoned out.

A Mysterious Blindness

Likewise, Samuel (ASC) described how his passion for photography left little room for much else:

I discovered photography ... and it became my obsession and unfortunately, I get most of the pleasure for my life from that and she doesn't share that ... I cannot give up what I love, she is unable to join me in it and therefore we've agreed to disagree on that, she does her thing and I do mine.

Therefore, an extreme focus can produce some positive outcomes regarding talents and expertise. Still, in the context of relationships, an extreme self-focus is not usually beneficial. When people are able to spend time on shared goals while having a mutual bigger picture for their relationship, it allows for the development of a more united, integrated and caring relationship.

Divided Notions

Due to their atypical cognitive abilities, people with ASC are less able to conceptualise themselves from another's perspective, are less able to distinguish between self and others, are less self-aware, have difficulty maintaining a stable self-concept, and can experience problems with adapting an unstable self-concept to ever-changing environments, such as relationships (Coutelle et al., 2020; Garon et al., 2022; Lyons & Fitzgerald, 2013). Without a good grasp on a sense of self, it is impossible to modify behaviour to suit the circumstances or relate to the needs of others. Additionally, the process of identifying with others is crucial for a normal development of the self-other association in relationships and is the basis for understanding and connecting with other minds.

Have We Gone Nuts?

A self-other overlap, (or including others in the self), is a psychological construct that emerges from people's motivation to form and maintain close relationships. It involves a sense of 'oneness' or 'interconnectedness' with close others. Research has suggested that a self-other overlap may be influenced by a host of relationship factors, such as shared experience, self-disclosure, or the motivation to draw another person closer to the self (Liu, 2014).

A strong sense of self-other overlap in relationships has been shown to increase prosocial behaviour (Feng et al., 2020; Liu, 2014), strengthen social bonds (Galinsky et al., 2005), develop unique, intimate links between people in relationships (Quintard et al., 2020), while also cultivating social closeness, forging lasting relationships and building complex understanding of others (Waugh & Fredrickson, 2006). Consequently, having a healthy self-other overlap plays an important role in maintaining relationships. However, due to the difficulties people on the spectrum have with social-emotional reciprocity and sharing thoughts and feelings, a healthy self-other overlap often becomes unattainable in neurodiverse relationships, as a sense of 'oneness' or 'interconnectedness' is difficult to achieve. Maggie's (NT) disappointment confirmed lower degrees of self-other overlap in her relationship:

> *He's happy with no or very little connection, he's quite content with it. So yeah, I'm not ... That disconnects us because I won't put myself forward anymore and share as much as I would like to share with him because of his reaction and his unknowing of how to deal with it on an emotional level.*

A Mysterious Blindness

Laura (NT) bemoaned this low level too:

I wish he paid me more attention, noticed me more, shared more of his inner life with me. Wish he'd share activities with me.

Wally's (ASC) regret revealed how his limitations were shaping lower levels of self-other overlap in his relationship:

Our relationship is kind of in some ways more like flatmates … She has said things like 'I'm not even sure whether you love me', so she obviously has an expectation of that but clearly, I'm not able to, even though I say it. I try and do things. I've obviously not been able to express that through support, so I think she has an expectation that will be through some kind of emotional support that I may even not recognise the need to give at the time she needs it. So yeah, it's a bit of a minefield.

Barry (ASC) shared his reasoning for a shortage of these factors in his relationship:

I suppose where there is not a lot of animosity going on simply because there's not a lot of interaction.

According to Weinstein et al. (2016), there are many benefits to a well-developed sense of self-other overlap. Individuals who feel a greater sense of self-other overlap in their close relationships, whether romantic, family or best friends, tend to experience a higher cognitive interdependence with the people in their close relationships, which promotes a more invested and intensely personal way of relating with them. A greater sense of self-other overlap is reflected in the blending of identity from 'I' to 'we' and 'many studies cite this as one important aspect of interpersonal closeness that is partly responsible for shared intimacy' (p. 130). People who identify as having high self-other overlap will maintain positive views of others in their relationships despite going through some unfavourable times. Lower self-other overlap in relationships can lead to having a tough time maintaining positive perceptions of significant others. Therefore, greater perceptions of overlap between the self and another introduces better relationship satisfaction, increases relationship commitment, improves the influences between boredom and a lower relationship satisfaction, and lowers relationship dissolution rates. Tracy (NT) revealed that the lower levels of self-other overlap in her relationship had triggered her own withdrawal:

*I do not seek to communicate much anymore. There are several reasons for this. Communication with him is not 'exciting'. Conversations fall flat and somehow are not kept alive. He gives me the impression he does not **want** to speak. Countless times he has walked away mid-sentence, often without having responded at all. Because I only found out about AS 3 years ago, it means that 21 years went by without my having any explanation of why this was the case. I thought he was being mean, stand-offish, proud, and that he was out to show me he didn't need or even want me in his life. With time, I just withdrew and lost interest in everything. He is an expert in giving monosyllabic answers when I am expecting a 'normal' answer of several extensive sentences. Sometimes I have to ask so many questions just to get a very basic piece of information, that anyone else would have given me immediately. I have told him time and time again that I am no wiser after one of his answers than before I asked the question.*

A Mysterious Blindness

An anonymous survey respondent (NT) disclosed a similar reaction:

I no longer have any expectations of the relationship and so this means fewer disappointments. There has been no intimacy for many years due to his lack of interest (not only in me but anyone), and so I requested some time ago that we sleep separately, which he complied to without argument! As my partner cannot determine what he wants out of our relationship I simply get on with my life independently for many things. I believe at this point we are together because it is financially viable for each of us!

While withdrawing from difficult situations may relieve some situations, when dealing with conflicting thoughts and emotions, another common strategy the psyche can use to avoid feeling anxiety is compartmentalisation. Compartmentalisation is a form of psychological defence mechanism in which thoughts and feelings are pushed down and kept separated or isolated from each other in the mind. This can happen when we feel cognitive dissonance (when we feel stressed because of conflicting thoughts, beliefs or attitudes) or when we have unpleasant feelings or experiences. To avoid cognitive dissonance, we may compartmentalise instead.

Compartmentalisation can be used in healthy or unhealthy ways. If used in moderation and combined with self-reflection and healthy emotional processing it can be an effective and valuable tool in stress management. It can, however, become a maladaptive coping strategy that prevents people from processing their negative experiences (Graham & Clark, 2006). This can be in relation to oneself or about others. It can be a conscious or an unconscious activity, which is used to avoid the unpleasant aspects of life. We may intentionally compartmentalise if we want to avoid feeling emotional pain or past trauma. However, by choosing (unconsciously or consciously) to avoid the source of our pain, we often create more difficulties for ourselves such as anxiety, discontentment, depression and unresolved grief, which can trigger other problems in our relationships.

When compartmentalisation is in relation to other people, they can be viewed unrealistically as totally defective at times and totally flawless at other times. This dualistic thinking naturally influences behaviour to fluctuate as well, resulting in a demonstration of affection when considering others as 'perfect' but becoming distant and aloof when others are considered 'imperfect'. When compartmentalisation is in relation to oneself, positive and negative knowledge about oneself is segregated into classes that remain distinct from each other. Focusing on positive attributes tends to build high self-esteem and positive mood, but focusing on negative attributes tends to produce low self-esteem and a negative mood (Showers & Zeigler-Hill, 2007). When fluctuating between two distinct behaviour patterns, it can appear to others as someone who has two distinct personalities, one kind and the other unkind, or commonly referred to as 'Jekyll and Hyde' (Graham & Clark, 2006). Georgia (NT) described the difficulties of living with her partner's compartmentalised thinking and related behaviour:

They learn to live in our world, they pick up on, they learn what is appropriate and what is not appropriate in certain social situations. I think that if they'd lived with a person for long enough, they learn how to manipulate them, and they'll use that skill to their advantage, and I think that is intentional. It's almost like a Jekyll and Hyde … you know you can see they have the potential to be kind and they're not always … but then they can flip and that's when the other side, it's almost like the other side of their brain is well, 'I need this right now so I'm going to do whatever it takes to have my needs fulfilled and if that means making that person back down these are the things that I'm going to say to that person'. That's intentional! And I think that's where I've had problems during counselling and just trying to deal with, 'Do I stay or do I go' … How do I communicate when he's being like that. That's not okay, or how do you even have the strength to keep going when that's what you're dealing with.

Likewise, Katy (NT) described the kind/mean contrasts she observed in Ronald (ASC):

He is very moody. Has massive mood swings and I would say that those mood swings seem to manifest as if he is on a high, and therefore he can get really, really silly as a wheel really, and quite childlike, and on a low and he gets very 'agro' and very anxious … He is very difficult, but he can be very charming, and people love, they love him. He meets new people, and they think he is fantastic, and I sit there and I think, 'You have no idea.' Hahaha. 'You have absolutely no idea.' And yet there are some sides to him that I really love. And when we are companionable, we are companionable. But that can change any second. So, it is a bit like treading on eggshells, living with him. And it's exhausting, and we battle all the time, and I will try to the best of my ability not to buy into an enraged discussion if you can call it that, but occasionally I just feel I've got to stand my ground and protect myself and I get very upset about the fact that he

*completely distorts the person I am … I certainly feel lonely
at times, because he lacks empathy and he is so argumentative
and he is such a know it all and yet there is this weird kind
of companionship that we have and I don't know whether it
is habit … and the terrifying prospect of leaving … it is not
an easy relationship at all … And I think sometimes they
do mean it. They have still got personality that dictates the
way, the way they do things.*

Renee (NT) revealed that while she understood that stress
activated Patrick's (ASC) Jekyll and Hyde behaviour, it meant
that she couldn't be 'herself':

*If he's highly stressed, no he doesn't hear a thing he's just off
and 'Bang!' Then saying that, that hasn't happened now for
well a little while … I don't feel able to like open myself up
again to being that emotional person with him because you
know it just comes back just like that and … it totally knocks
you for six and … I think 'How can you be so horrible?'…
It's weird, it's weird, it's weird.*

On the other hand, due to an inability to talk with others
about the ASC-NT difficulties, Rae (NT) defined her life as
split into two separate compartments:

*He said, 'It is kind of fun fighting all the time.' I said, 'You've
got to be bloody joking', because it's miserable for me. I mean
he can't, he must be miserable as well … and it just like, I'm
not a nice person when I am around him either, it changes
you doesn't it? You sort of live in this Jekyll and Hyde sort
of life too when you are with your girlfriends and stuff …
cause when they see him socially, they say 'Oh, everybody
loves Isaac'… 'What do you fight about?' and I thought, 'I*

can't even begin to tell you.' I can't even put it into words because that sort of interaction doesn't happen when you are out socially.

Research has confirmed that the partners and family members of those who display compartmentalised thinking find it hard to deal with a person whose view of them fluctuates between positive and negative. Predictability is a crucial component of interpersonal trust but 'instability in how one is viewed and treated by a partner is likely to contribute to decreased relationship satisfaction' (Graham & Clark, 2006, p. 663). Georgia (NT) described these difficulties:

What I noticed about my husband is he can say he has Asperger's. He can acknowledge that there's an issue, but the willingness to put the work in to adapt his behaviours so that he could live within his family was not there. By comparison when I thought I was going crazy, I was like I have to, my family and my marriage is way too important for me to destroy it, I want to be well, I want to be a mother and a wife whereas he's kind of like, 'Well I've got Asperger's so I'm off the hook now', and whilst he knows that there's literature out there, because ... he reads scientific papers so he understands the intellectual level so he knows that the issue is there but I think ... to really work at it and to really try and change and be prepared to say 'Okay Ross, when you do stuff like that, that's not okay', and to be able to accept and hear that and say 'Oh okay, she may be right in this situation'. I don't think he'll ever let me say that to him. There's not that willingness to say, 'That's not okay'.

By compartmentalising to avoid dealing with the difficulties that come our way, we run the risk of becoming overwhelmed, angry, emotionally unavailable, shut down or else people pleasing as we become disconnected from our own self and our authentic truth and needs. Feelings and emotions, no matter how overwhelming or worrying they may seem, are important indicators of what is going on inside of us. Pushing them down only tends to make navigating and managing them harder, if not impossible. However, since the typical ways to manage emotions are often more difficult for those on the spectrum, they may be more disposed towards developing compartmentalised thinking. Katy (NT) suggested that those on the spectrum use compartmentalised behaviour as a way to comfort themselves:

> *The emotional stuff. Yeah. Yeah, I mean to me, from where I stand … I just can't believe that it is anything but 'This is going to cause a lot of emotional upheaval. I am going to remove myself from it.' And once they have removed themselves from it and felt safe, because I have observed my grandson, he will go into a safe place. He has got these little hidey-holes that he likes to go into, when there is an emotional, when he has been really badly behaved, and we have been looking after him, he will disappear … He has gone to his little safe place, and he says 'Leave me alone. I am in my safe place.' And you leave him alone and he will come out when he is ready and it will be like nothing has ever happened, because in a way he has comforted himself. So, I think, as an adult, an Aspie adult maybe, is forgetting, deliberately shutting down … in order to comfort themselves.*

In contrast to compartmentalised mental processes, possessing an integrative self-structure (i.e. unified reasoning) enables individuals to hold both positive and negative self-beliefs concurrently. An integrative self-structure allows individuals to maintain a balanced mood, and their overall feelings about self and others are viewed realistically as having both strengths and weaknesses that sometimes provide support and at other times need to be supported (Graham & Clark, 2006). People with unified reasoning remain more stable, have greater realism and moderated self-views, and possibly have increased resilience. They tend to feel accepted by others, which is an antidote to fearful feelings in regard to how others view them (Showers & Zeigler-Hill, 2007).

Whether compartmentalised mental processes are in regard to oneself or in regard to others, they are unstable over time. Connected to mood and self-esteem, compartmentalised reasoning will naturally oscillate as life experiences change, creating unpredictable behaviour (Showers & Zeigler-Hill, 2007). This unpredictability may create instability within relationships. When compartmentalised mental processes or behaviour is combined with unrecognised or unaccepted autism, it can set up destructive patterns within relationships, strengthening some of the unconventional aspects of these relationships. It may follow that when people on the spectrum possess a more integrative self-structure and are able to accept themselves in light of recognition of a diagnosis; their relationship may have a greater likelihood of success.

Support Thoughts

To provide appropriate support and understanding to people in neurodiverse relationships, it is important to understand the cognitive mechanisms underlying the internalising and externalising difficulties that influence the actions of those on the autism spectrum and how these impact on them and those who live with and love them. Once understanding of these aspects occur, it will provide a framework to better support people in these relationships. Yet, since most of this conduct occurs behind closed doors, professionals, family or friends will rarely, if at all, observe any of these behaviours. Therefore, the development of targeted supports and interventions will only be possible when taking into account the stories of all those involved.

The next chapter continues the discussion on the cognitive mechanisms underlying some of the brain differences between the two groups of people and the impact that these differences have on each.

4

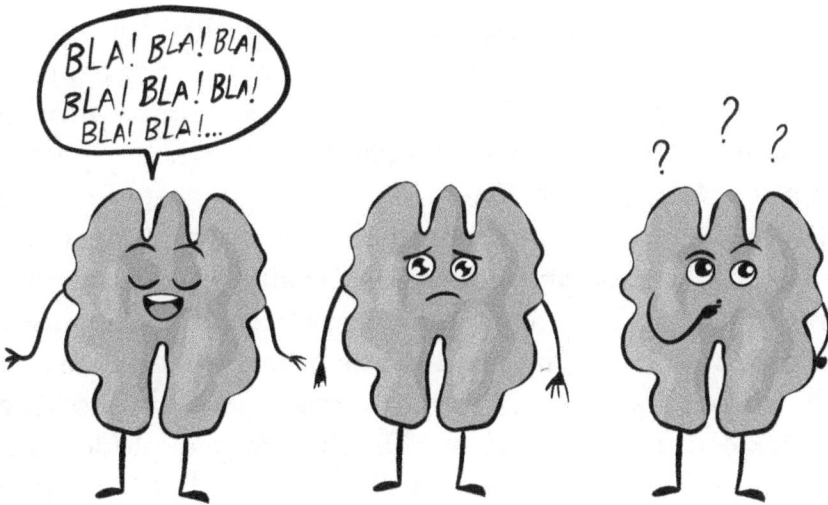

Associated
Anomalies

Have We Gone Nuts?

**'Hell, in my opinion, is never finding your true
self and never living your own life or knowing
who you are.'**
John Bradshaw

Due to their different cognitive and self-awareness abilities, adults with ASC often experience difficulties with understanding what others are thinking or feeling, regularly get anxious about social situations, generally find it difficult to socialise and mostly find it challenging when expected to say how they feel. They may overcompensate for their difficulties by talking too much. They may experience anxiety, low mood and feelings of despair from their various interaction malfunctions, sometimes becoming depressed as a result. They may experience a heightened sense of confusion, sometimes becoming blunt, rude or showing a lack of interest in others. Or, they may explode with aggressive outburst behaviours, often without intending to do so.

According to Ozsivadjian et al. (2021), 'there is emerging empirical support for a number of socio-cognitive mechanisms being implicated in the development and maintenance of high rates of internalising and externalising difficulties in ASC' (p. 715). These internalising behaviours (anxiety and low mood) and externalising behaviours (aggressive or outburst behaviours, and irritability) in autism are very common responses to the frustrations and inabilities to make headway in their relationships. However, the attempts of others to understand and compensate for these challenging reactions can be a complicated, demanding task as well.

Associated Anomalies

Understanding that these internalising and externalising difficulties are often triggered by attempts to compensate for the different cognitive mechanisms in ASC is essential for developing targeted supports and interventions, both for those with autism and their partners and family members.

A Matter of Monologues

It is well known that the differences in neurology for autistic people triggers difficulties with reciprocal conversation. An aspect of that difficulty is the unstructured nature of face-to-face conversation and the need to coordinate other modes of communication, such as eye gaze with speech. To compensate for this difficulty, adults with ASC will often stick to topics of their own interest which gives rise to a more monologue-style of speech (Nadig et al., 2010). However, engaging in frequent one-sided conversations in a relationship will often add to struggles with reciprocal conversation.

Additionally, combining conversational difficulties with the engrossing nature of circumscribed interests (i.e. intense preoccupation with a specific interest) may strengthen a tendency for perseveration. The term perseveration is used to describe any continuation, or recurrence of an activity without an appropriate stimulus (i.e. continuing to talk on about a topic after the conversation has moved on to other topics).

Research shows that perseveration continues throughout the lifespan of people with ASC, however it is a problematic distractor to others and can be a source of stigma (Arora, 2012). This type of monologue may further the difficulties they have with interacting, and sometimes, may lead to causing unintended offense. Dana (NT) shared how her son tended to perseverate on topics that others found a bit awkward:

When you talk to him it's a very forced eye contact, if you're not talking to him, he will not engage … he won't listen and hear where he can fit into a conversation and jump in. He stays off to the side and manages to focus on some object or something and then somebody has to get him and bring him in, and once you've done that then he turns the conversation into what he wants to talk about … in his case it's a very extreme religion so it's very off-putting to other people in the room because nobody really expected that so it's just odd.

Perseveration and the susceptibility toward running commentaries can overshadow conversations, making it difficult to discuss any other topics. Beth (NT) described how she had to take charge of a conversation when Christopher (ASC) became perseverative:

Sometimes … he can get onto the one topic and just go on and on and on and I'll have to change the subject. I'll have to say, 'Now look I've got to discuss this with you, it's really important.'

Lucy (NT) also shared the challenges of managing her ASC partner's tendency for monologues in conversations:

Bear in mind he loves talking to me about what he wants to talk about. He's going overseas shortly … so he's itching to tell me about it, all the time and when I walked away from him a while ago and sort of said, 'Look it's either, it is the psychologist or nothing.' I said 'I've now got to start looking after me. This is going nowhere. We can never have a proper relationship or anywhere part near one unless you're willing to learn some strategies to deal with this, so I'm going to walk away and realistically I don't want you to call me.' ... 'Oh well, you've made up your mind then. I won't cop an ultimatum.'... but then he did phone ... because he's itching to tell me all about an update on this Europe trip he's doing, so he doesn't really want me, that much I do know, but I've just got to keep him at arm's length and say, 'No, no.'

An anonymous survey respondent (NT) mentioned a negative outcome of her partner's monologues:

Holding conversations are always one-sided and usually end with forgiveness/compromise, but never resolved.

Snared by Sorrow

Perseveration is also known to be triggered by stress and anxiety and feeling stressed and anxious are common experiences for people with autism. So common, in fact that it is now recognised that there is an association between autism and anxiety, with estimations of approximately 80 percent of autistic people feeling mildly anxious practically every day for most of their life. Sometimes, they can experience consistent and severe anxiety in particular situations, such as when there are changes in routine or expectations, uncertainty in what to do or what is going to happen, fear of limitations and making mistakes, or undesirable feelings related to specific sensory experiences.

Research has confirmed that an anxiety disorder is the most common mental health problem for autistic adults

(Hwang et al., 2020). It has been found that sometimes, the level of anxiety experienced may be perceived as more disabling than the diagnostic characteristics of autism. As reported in Book 1, participants with ASC described many instances of anxiety. A fear of failure, the complexities of emotional conversation, and multiple experiences of malfunctioned communications were reported to be the main motivations behind feelings of anxiety, stress and a sense of powerlessness. Sandra (ASC) explained why some conversations caused her to feel anxious:

> If it's not emotional … it's easier to have a conversation about it. Emotional ones I start to kind of think what I should be doing or what the other person wants me to be saying and trying to really understand and listen to the other person, because I know it's an important thing at that moment … I have to be more mindful of the connection between us at the moment and what I'm doing and if that seems okay in the situation and there's more thought about my actions and my words … because I think I'm more kind of anxious about me saying the right thing.

Beth (NT) explained that sometimes she needs to take the blame to manage Christopher's (ASC) anxiety:

> If it's become unproductive, I'll just say, 'Look I think we're going to have to talk about this again later, we're not going anywhere at the moment.' If he's too far gone in his anxiety, then we'll have to keep nutting it out and sometimes I'll just go, 'Okay. You're right. I'm wrong. I'm the idiot here. We'll just leave it.' But that's when his anxiety is really ramped up, yeah.

Associated Anomalies

Renee (NT) noted that Patrick (ASC) relied on scripts to deal with his stress:

When he's particularly stressed, he'll go back to the script which is this one that he's got and no matter how you try and kind of change that or talk to him about it or whatever, it just keeps coming back, it's the same old stuff.

When asked how she dealt with it, she answered:

What I do, again it depends on the level of his anxiety and if I notice, you've just got to take all the emotion out of it, you can't be upset about something. I can't talk to him if I was upset about something because he just doesn't cope with that, so I have learned that I take the emotion out of it, be very clear about what I want to say and if he's really stressed I won't talk about it until a day or two later which again I know is not ideal but that's how it is really.

Stress and anxiety have been shown to be associated with depression. Many autistic people report lower feelings of self-worth, express fewer positive traits about themselves, internalise problems, struggle with negative self-focused thoughts, tend to experience symptoms of anxiety and depression, worry in social situations, encounter feelings of sadness and hopelessness, and as a result, often lack motivation (Burrows et al., 2017).

Both perseveration and depression are somewhat common in ASC (Keenan et al., 2018). The propensity to perseverate in the ASC population, when linked with depression can lead to rumination. Rumination is a maladaptive form of emotion processing which involves perseverative thoughts that revolve around negative emotions or situations (Patel et al., 2017). Rumination can cause you to remain focused on the cause of your frustrations, stresses or anxieties. When asked how she dealt with difficult conversations between her and her partner, Stella (ASC) confirmed this connection:

I ruminate on them, which often causes further stress.

Since rumination is a passive dwelling upon what is distressing, past mistakes, regrets or shortcomings, it can prevent the mind turning to positive thoughts. It can also prevent problem-solving because the emotional distress remains the focus and not in finding solutions. Jim (ASC) shared how his conversations with Dianne (NT) did not produce the results that he wanted, and his resulting frustration led to a negative belief pattern:

I try to get back to the point and facts … and compare it to whatever happened previously, or whatever you have done previously … I think, on my side of it, I just get so frustrated and upset, I just don't even bother talking to her. It's just like falling on deaf ears, and she will make a comment that 'You don't listen to me'… but neither does she listen to me, so it makes it a bit hard. But in reality if the environment is, where we are trying to interact, we are either yelling, or she doesn't listen, where she will explain, 'Well there is a typical example of your behaviour'… makes me very depressed. Got to a stage where I think, 'What's the use of bloody living in this environment?' … at some stages … I thought I may as well just jump off a cliff, but it is … very depressing. You know you're trying to have a conversation … She said, 'Well you should try', and I'm thinking, 'But try at what?'

Associated Anomalies

On the other hand, Dianne revealed how Jim's inability to understand what she was trying to convey led to her own negative feelings and apathy:

I'm just tired of the pushing now, so often when the message doesn't get through, I will either lose it, which is not the way to go, and I find that only makes him withdraw all the more and I know that, but I just think, well who cares. So, I will go right off, or I just don't bother.

When Wanda (NT) was asked why she had answered in her survey that she felt powerless to discuss difficulties with Wally (ASC), she said:

Yeah because of the issues with his depression he went through where if anything troubling came up … he would get very emotional, he would sort of like, not angry, he would break down basically and have to go … like take himself away from the situation and he would end up going to our room, shutting the door and fall asleep for hours. I guess it was sort of avoidant, but it was also that state of depression where he couldn't deal with things … I think that was some kind of conditioning to me that I can't, don't want to bring up things that might sort of end up in that situation, I suppose. So that's really hard.

Nora (NT) also lamented her (ASC) partner's helplessness:

Hopeless, helpless, they're helpless.

An anonymous survey respondent (NT) described the devastating results of a son's depression:

Have We Gone Nuts?

My Asperger son (26) has high anxiety levels at the moment and can be very hard to decide what sort of mood he wakes up in and this can change the mood of the whole day. However, I persist and try to get a feel of the mood for the day and do not try to intrude on his space. But I feel that this can cause things to stagnate and not find a mutually acceptable time to discuss important issues of how he can progress and cope with the depression. This causes me a lot of frustration as I know that, if left, his depression may escalate into him feeling worthless and may cause him to self-harm. I am almost at my wits end to getting help with my adult son – every resource I have tried are unreliable and don't get back to you with follow-up help!

Many ASC participants confirmed their partner's attitudes, sharing that they felt conversations with their NT partners were not worth the effort because they were doomed to fail:

STELLA   *I don't know what to say … I feel it's in vain, that nothing would really change, that for every complaint I make, I receive three accusations.*

EDITH   *I just don't feel like I can create a situation where he's pulled back … with regard to things that he's already got a stated opinion on and so, you just don't have any sense of certainty that you can make headway on it, and I mean you can have a sort of hopeless feeling around that … I feel if I wanted to raise something that I can, I just don't ever have the chance to do it, because it can only go in the direction that he's already thought and decided on and that's just a foregone conclusion which isn't a particularly successful start. Well, you know you feel like you're never going to make any progress.*

DANIEL *There are a great many ways in which conversation can go wrong, and I'm adept at more than a few of them. All too easily I can slip into silence, become unpleasantly garrulous, or just say the wrong thing.*

SAMUEL *Yeah, with regard to a lot of things I probably respond in a way that most people would think impractical and so I have most of my life. My responses to those sorts of conversations are disregarded because of that, so I'm used to it in a sense, but the things that I think of first come to mind in response to certain issues or whatever else are considered impractical by those that I'm speaking with.*

It appears that feeling helpless may be a core feature of ASC. The presence of persistent and enduring feelings of helplessness seems to be very common. However, it is often an invisible ordeal, both to those with intimate knowledge of the person, and in many instances, to those with ASC themselves. Feelings of helplessness arises when thinking that bad outcomes are brought about by one's own actions whereas good outcomes are the result of other causes. In essence, one feels helpless to make good things occur, unable to prevent bad things from happening and ruminating on the assumption that this lack of control is permanent. Research has shown conclusively that the brain is a plastic living organ, that it can change itself and that exposure to new and different ways of thinking has the ability to change brain structure and function (Doidge, 2007).

However, since rumination can keep people stuck in negative thinking and prevent an ability to evaluate something or someone in a different way, it can maintain feelings of helplessness. Anger rumination can also result. Anger rumination is repetitive thoughts and persistent dwelling on anger-provoking events, which can increase anger, worry and negative emotions. Research has found that it is common for people on the spectrum to experience high levels of anger rumination (Ibrahim et al., 2019; Patel et al., 2017; Pugliese et al., 2014). Research also suggests that there may be a link between anger rumination and depression in autistic adults, although the understanding of this relationship is still evolving. Given that adults with ASC can experience challenges in regulating emotions, including anger, anger rumination may exacerbate these difficulties and potentially contribute to the development or maintenance of depressive symptoms. When Jim (ASC) was asked how he felt about the communication difficulties between them, he answered:

Oh, again, disagreements, hurt, disappointment, just makes things very uncomfortable. Yeah, hurt, disappointment, loneliness, depression, yeah. That's the way I feel most times but, can't do too much about it. So that's the way it is, that's the way the cookie crumbles.

The co-occurrence of anger rumination and depression can have a significant impact on the overall wellbeing and quality of life of autistic adults and those around them. It may lead to increased social difficulties, impaired daily functioning and reduced psychological wellbeing. Research on this topic is still limited, and more studies are needed to better understand the specific mechanisms underlying the relationship between anger rumination and depression in autistic adults. Nonetheless, recognising the potential connection can help inform interventions and support strategies aimed at improving emotional wellbeing in this population.

It is important to note that many autistic adults can regularly experience cyclical feelings of sadness and pessimism that can develop into a clinical depression. According to Williams et al. (2021) a major depressive disorder is exceedingly common in adults on the spectrum 'with an estimated 23% current prevalence and 37% lifetime prevalence in this population' (p. 858). Feelings of loneliness, not being understood or valued by others, the social isolation or else exhaustion due to socialising, trying to manage or suppress emotions and coping with sensory sensitivities are many of the reasons as to why an autistic person may become sad and depressed.

While some adults with ASC may exhibit classic symptoms of depression, such as persistent sadness, loss of interest in activities, changes in appetite or sleep patterns, and feelings of worthlessness, others may demonstrate atypical symptoms, such as increased irritability, meltdowns, or heightened sensitivity to sensory stimuli. Georgia (NT) thought that it could also be a trust issue:

And they have to trust their partner, that's the issue that my husband has with me is that he didn't trust me that I was in it for his benefit, that I wanted to help him. I wasn't going to do it for him, but I wanted him to be able to adapt so that he could stay in our relationship. I don't think he trusted that my intentions were not pure … so I think sometimes it's a trust issue and that goes back to these Aspie's being really fearful, they seem to be really fearful, and my daughter said, 'I think Dad's convinced that, he believes that we conspire against him. We conspire to make his life miserable, we set out to make his life miserable', and she said 'I believe that that's what he thinks', and some of the things he's said I'm inclined to think that he does think that, that I deliberately set out to make his life miserable and you're like no! Your life's miserable because we don't get on.

Wally's (ASC) conversation confirmed some of the things that Georgia had discussed. He lamented the fear and feelings of hopelessness that held him back from resolving disagreements with Wanda (NT), which instead, led him to self-protecting behaviours and a cautious, evasive approach to interactions with her:

It's a scary place to go … so I will avoid … it's avoiding that confrontation … and then she says, 'You'll go silent for a couple of hours and then … you'll talk about stuff like as if nothing has happened' … and I'm like 'Well what else am I supposed to do?'… Maybe it was unresolved, but we can't keep hammering away at something until it's resolved because some of these things are unresolvable.

Many of the difficulties that autistic adults experience can lead to a confusing set of circumstances within relationships. Recognising that depression may underpin some behaviours is crucial for the overall wellbeing of those with autism, their partners and family members, and for their relationships.

Captured by Confusion

Unsurprisingly, all relationships have their moments of confusion and misunderstandings. However, when including an inability to interpret the non-verbal cues of loved ones, this autistic shortcoming may pave the way for even more confusing events to occur.

Typically, when people perceive a discrepancy between the verbal and non-verbal signals that someone is relaying, they tend to base their judgement on the non-verbal information they are observing, rather than the verbal information that they are hearing (Pelzl et al., 2022). Research has found people typically tend to have more belief in the non-verbal cues they see rather than what is actually said because verbal communication is a deliberate act and is much easier to manipulate, whereas body language, facial expressions and vocal characteristics are not so easy to control (Pelzl et al., 2022). As a result, recognising emotional states correctly is highly important for successful social interaction. When non-verbal signals are consistent with the words said, it increases trust, clarity and rapport (Pelzl et al., 2022). However, inaccurate perception of nonverbal emotional cues contributes to misunderstanding and difficulties in social interactions.

Since people with ASC experience difficulties with interpreting the non-verbal signals of others, there is a high likelihood of inaccurate reading of the emotional cues of their partners and family members. This may contribute to many of the misunderstandings that occur between them and may also increase a sense of confusion between them. Many participants described how they attempted to get through the resulting difficulties. Sophie (NT) shared that being direct worked for her:

I had to learn to be direct and to the point when asking for things or conveying a need of mine ... given AS partners are not great at picking up on hints or those slight emotional clues, we NTs give off.

Similarly, Rose (NT) expressed a need to be direct:

There's been times where I try to be affectionate ... I won't realise that a touch is unexpected by him ... he doesn't see it and then it's a surprise to him and then he has a startled response and ... where most people they feel it coming, and he really doesn't and ... sometimes I'm like, 'I was just trying to give you a hug, like what the hec?' ... but at first, I wasn't really putting out ... clear verbal communication because I didn't know ... he couldn't read the tiny little signals that I was putting out so ... that was a lot to navigate ... now if I want more affection I just literally say, 'I want you to affect me', and then he gives me a hug or something ha, ha.

Whereas Diana (NT) described some of the impacts on her:

I suppose for my husband subtle things you can do just kind of go straight over his head, and there is a bit of lack of I suppose of caring for even the needs or wants of somebody else. It does seem that he's quite self-centred a lot of the time but I'm sure he doesn't really mean to be, he's really got quite a nice nature underneath it all, but sometimes I suppose you can take it personally because it comes across kind of a bit callous or insensitive but yeah he doesn't mean to be.

Associated Anomalies

Nora (NT) explained that she was learning to accept her partner's inability to read her cues:

The other day I reached out, and we were having a conversation and we laughed, and I just lent my cheek over for him to kiss me and he just sort of didn't even notice that I'd lent, didn't even notice, whereas in the past I would have gone, 'Oh you've pulled away from me, what's wrong with you?' Whereas now, I'm just like 'Oh wow, he just didn't even pick up that cue.'

On the other hand, Murray (ASC) gave his assessment on the reasons that lie beneath:

I think it's just that miscommunication on the language we use in terms of the way I think through something logically and explain it logically versus a non-Asperger person to think about it more intuitively and more the subtlety of the differences. Whereas I'm 1+2=3 and very black and white, factual logical steps, and to them they might look quite complex but they're still logical steps, whereas I will miss the little subtleties in explanation. If Jane explains something to me or tells something to me, if there's subtleties within it that aren't explained, I will miss them and then that can often change the overall meaning of the conversation, and even things like body language and the tone of voice and that sort of stuff, hence I sort of miss. I pick it up certainly better with my wife than anyone else because I know from experience if she's shying left or looking a certain way then that means something but that's because I've spent 20 years with her and see her every day, I can pick up on those things, but certainly subtleties from other people, and even a lot of her subtleties, I miss.

The autistic intolerance of uncertainty (Rodgers et al., 2018) has the power to strengthen confusing situations in neurodiverse relationships. Intolerance of uncertainty is the tendency to react negatively to uncertain situations and events on an emotional, cognitive and behavioural level (Ozsivadjian et al., 2021). It is well known that people on the spectrum often find uncertain situations stressful and upsetting as they have a tendency to interpret ambiguous information as threatening and commonly find it difficult to function in the face of uncertainty. An intolerance of uncertainty can also heighten internalising behaviours such as feelings of helplessness and depression and externalising behaviours such as withdrawal, anxious agitation and irritability or aggression and outburst behaviours.

It is now becoming understood that these behaviours bear a conceptual resemblance to the restricted and repetitive behaviours that people with autism routinely exhibit, such as insistence on sameness, inflexible adherence to routines and difficulty tolerating change. Evidence is now emerging that intolerance of uncertainty has a central role in the relationship between ASC and anxiety since uncertainty is stressful and upsetting and not knowing what is going to happen is considered negative, and consequently, should be avoided at all costs (Rodgers et al., 2018). These difficulties, compounded by the problems autistic people have with holding back a current idea and flexibly switching to another idea, may also contribute to less flexible coping strategies to manage difficult emotions. As a result, internalised difficulties such as feelings of helplessness and depression, as well as externalised problems such as aggression, outburst behaviours and irritability can be heightened. Georgia (NT) discussed what happened when Ross (ASC) had to contend with the uncertainty of her emotional responses:

> *They get fearful because they're frightened that if they upset you, you're going to get angry and then they can't deal with your anger ... so they don't say anything or they themselves respond with anger or they shut down and they retreat ... communication just breaks down.*

Tracy (NT) described the unexpected hostilities that resulted from the uncertainty a new baby brings to a household:

> *When we had our first child, James did not seem to accept him. He was in a terrible mood all the time, and never did anything with the baby. Sometimes he would not touch the baby for days. Communication was like war.*

Winnie (NT) understood that anxiety underpinned her husband's need to control his environment:

> *If I do something and it may not be in a logical sequential order and he observes it, he will have to correct me and tell me, 'This is how you do it' and I will try and say, 'But we both reach the same end result, I just do it differently'. He has great frustration in that, having to cope with something that he sees as just manifestly wrong so he can't acknowledge that the end result's the same, it's the fact that I haven't followed the procedure that's correct ... It might be doing the dishes, it might be cooking something ... and he will get highly frustrated very quickly if I don't immediately do it the way he thinks it should be done ... but now I have to bite my tongue or just accept that ... it*

is more about his anxiety, [his] need to control it by things being a certain way.

Sophie (NT) described how an uncertain time of leaving on a road trip resulted in her partner having a meltdown:

A road trip we were to go on, he had it in his head we were going to depart by car no later than 8 am without telling me this. I worked the night before, and I needed to wash laundry for myself and this trip, pack, and prep the cat's stuff as well as the house before we departed … He had a mini meltdown when he asked me what was the latest time I would be ready, me stating 10 am. His response meltdown was, well we should just stay home now. There is no point in going (8-hour road trip to his brother's house where there was no deadline or appointed time to arrive). From my perspective he asked me what time, I told him, then he lost it on me, being grouchy and acting tantrummy. He failed to communicate his expectations with time. He will often do this to me when it comes to planning of trips and time-related things. I just have to prepare myself. Ironically, he said his father was the same way. By discussing the time issues, he had a few 'ah ha' moments and realised his father was an Aspie as well.

Whereas Rachelle (ASC) described the insecurities she felt about relationships:

I've never experienced anything else, so this is just what relationships are to me, full of misunderstandings and expectations that I have no idea what they expect.

Alexithymia is another difficulty that affects about 10% of the general population but about 50% of autistic adults and has been implicated in a range of internalising difficulties (Ozsivadjian et al., 2021). Reported in more detail in Book 1, alexithymia is described as a pronounced difficulty in identifying emotions, describing one's own emotions, and also communicating about emotions (Wilkinson, 2016). Alexithymia can have an adverse effect on abilities to emotionally connect with others (Eid & Boucher, 2012; Montebarocci et al., 2011). When an individual with autism has alexithymia, it can present as an added difficulty to inhibiting the meaningful conversation and essential giving and receiving of emotional language that are fundamental for relationship health. In Book 1, many ASC participants explained that expressing their feelings and emotions was extremely difficult, sometimes an insurmountable hurdle, and so it was something to be avoided at all costs. However, Wally (ASC) shared his awareness of the difficulty and attempts to triumph over it:

So, I'm aware of alexithymia, I'm definitely an autistic person who also is alexithymic and trying to identify what the feeling is and how to deal with it is really hard and it gets in the way of rationality. It gets in the way of progress in that. Yes, it's a tough place to go and although I want to go there, I recognise the need to go there, it f**ks me up.

Both groups of participants described high levels of frustration as they tried to work through the consistent confusion their differences caused. Maggie (NT) shared a frequent experience of the NT partner or family member; an inability to comprehend what was going on:

I couldn't define it. When Luke had left, I was trying to define the line of 'Is this him or is this the AS that's talking here?' I wasn't sure and it was really hard to define any kind of line of whether it's them or whether it's part of the AS, whether they can change, whether they can't change, whether they can make a decision and work on this, or they can't work on this, or all that kind of stuff. It does your head in.

On the other hand, Mary (ASC) described the confusion they both felt:

Alex can only act on the information that I give him and if I don't know it myself, and I'm behaving in a way that Alex is going 'You are saying this, but you are behaving like that. Do you really understand what you are dealing with?' And I will go, 'I've got no f**king clue ... I don't know what I am doing or feeling.'

Rae (NT) lamented this continual frustration and confusion:

They just tip you over the edge with the frustration and the annoyance and I just think 'Why is this so hard ... Everybody else can understand me ... you just get so confused when I try to talk.' ... People have got no idea, have they?

Sharon (ASC) described how she confused other people:

It confused them when I start to talk to them about my problems. I am also usually the most rational person among people I know, and their highly emotional reaction toward my problem can be very ineffective for me.

Malcolm (ASC) described the confusion he felt when trying to process conversations:

Associated Anomalies

She is trying to talk to me about an aspect of our relationship, what I hear is noise and yelling and confusion, so I have to go away and process it. And then she will follow me and will talk more, and it is like 'No, no, no, no!'

Whereas Murray (ASC) said talking together did help him and his wife overcome some of the confusion:

I do see things differently. Sometimes, we have miscommunication where she thinks the situation means X and I think it means Y and if we don't talk it through then we're not on the same page and there can be issues of confusion. But we find if we talk, we understand and I can explain the way I see it and often she will explain to me why that's not the way most people would see it, but at least we're talking through it.

Similarly, Phil (ASC) was trying to find ways to work through the confusion:

I don't communicate properly with her, no, because I find forming sentences and words very hard ... Well up to about a year or so ago, it used to just make me freeze and I couldn't think. I couldn't do anything because everything was happening too fast and everybody needed answers, and things needed to happen and I wasn't able to do anything, so I can't think. That's how it affects me, and it affects Robyn, she gets frustrated because she is not getting any assistance or help from me in the situation. I am slowly learning to be a bit better at that and not freeze and just say 'Woo, I need time to think, I need time to catch up.' I have learned how to do that.

115

Have We Gone Nuts?

An anonymous survey respondent (NT) described the rollercoaster ride of confusion:

Misunderstandings and confusions abound. [My] partner's delight in analysing communication breakdowns for an hour plus is exasperating – 'But I thought you ...' Insistence on maintaining a routine despite changed circumstances is highly challenging. Assigning a time and place and topic for important conversations, as in a meeting, has been helpful. Prior agreement guarantees attention, etc. My using the template 'When you ... I feel ...' was a turning point in the relationship.

When considering the cognitive theories, cognitive inflexibility and different self-awareness abilities discussed in the previous chapter, together with the behaviours discussed in this chapter, such as a tendency for perseveration and all its associated difficulties, intolerance of uncertainty and alexithymia, it is vital to understand that people in neurodiverse relationships often exist in a state of confusion, turmoil and insecurity.

Research is only at the beginning of understanding how these mechanisms function together to bring about some of the difficulties seen in neurodiverse relationships. Only when our understanding of these aspects improve and we begin to appreciate how the interactions between these mechanisms and the internalising/externalising difficulties seen in ASC, as well as the differing impacts on all involved in neurodiverse relationships, will it be possible to develop more effective and targeted interventions (Ozsivadjian et al., 2021).

Support Thoughts

The complex social, cognitive and affective divide between the two groups of people in neurodiverse relationships are revealed through the participants words in these studies. Their stories provide a comprehensive framework for understanding the contrasting difficulties and resulting impacts on each within these relationships.

Not only do their stories improve understanding of the day-to-day lives of those in neurodiverse relationships, but they also improve the potential for the development of targeted supports and interventions.

The next chapter discusses some of the consequences of these different cognitive mechanisms on each in a neurodiverse relationship. Also discussed are the resulting impacts on each of some of the internalising and externalising difficulties that autistic people can experience.

5

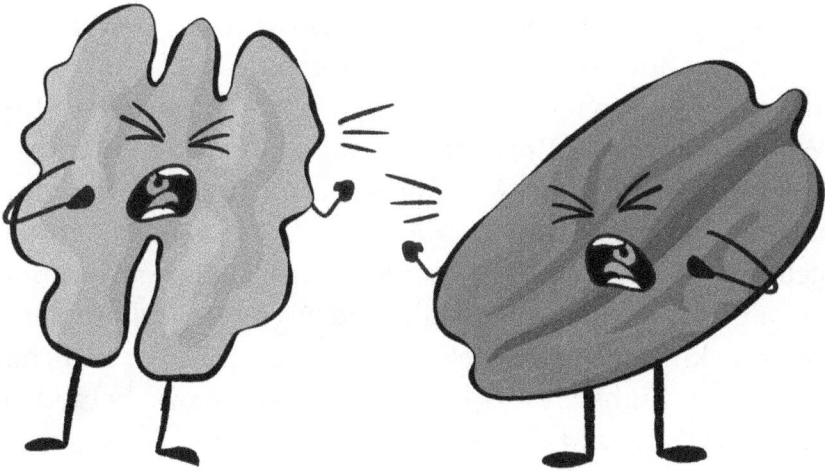

A Toxic Tailspin

Have We Gone Nuts?

'Just because it is explainable,
doesn't mean it's excusable.'
Anonymous

Several studies have reported that lower levels of adaptive behaviour among people with autism can contribute to greater symptoms of the internalising behaviours, such as anxiety and low mood, and externalising behaviours, such as aggressive or outburst behaviours and irritability (Woodman et al., 2016). Low adaptive behaviour in autism refers to difficulties or challenges in acquiring and applying practical skills necessary for daily life. These challenges often include common autistic difficulties, such as communication and language skills, social skills and cognitive and problem-solving skills. However, Woodman et al. (2016) found that possessing higher levels of adaptive behaviour helped to reduce anxious and depressed behaviours.

Interestingly, the study by Woodman et al. (2016) also discovered that maternal criticism or warmth were key factors in risk toward low adaptive behaviours or else protection from low adaptive behaviours in children with autism. In other words, there was a correlation between high levels of maternal criticism in early life and high symptoms of internalising and externalising difficulties in adults with autism. Likewise, there was a correlation between maternal warmth in early life and low symptoms. High symptoms of internalising and externalising difficulties may also increase potentials to experience meltdowns.

A Toxic Tailspin

Matters of Meltdown

It is well known that many autistic people experience meltdowns. A meltdown is an intense response to overwhelming sensory, emotional or environmental stimuli (Lewis & Stevens, 2023). It happens when someone becomes completely overwhelmed by their current situation, temporarily loses control of their behaviour and then finds it very hard to calm themselves. This loss of control can be expressed verbally, physically, or both. Similar to other commonplace autistic behaviour, meltdowns are often kept hidden behind closed doors. Meltdowns may increase the unconventional quality to these relationships, but they can be very hard to explain to others outside of the home.

There can be many different reasons for a meltdown. Sensory overload can be a significant trigger for meltdowns due to being overwhelmed by sensory stimuli such as loud noises, bright lights, strong smells or textures. This can lead to increased agitation, anxiety or discomfort. Withdrawal or shutdown can be another response to overwhelming situations, resulting in becoming unresponsive, non-communicative, or seeking isolation as a means of self-regulation and self-protection. Self-stimulatory behaviours can serve as a way to self-soothe or regulate sensory input and can include repetitive movements (e.g. rocking, leg tapping, hand-flapping), vocalisations or other self-comforting actions. In extreme cases of a meltdown, aggression towards others or else self-injurious behaviour which involves hitting, scratching, biting, or other injurious actions can develop. It's important to note that these behaviours are not intentional but can be a result of overwhelming emotions and sensory overload. It is also important to differentiate between meltdowns and intentional misbehaviour or temper tantrums. Autistic meltdowns are not deliberate acts of defiance but are rather a response to overwhelming circumstances (Lewis & Stevens, 2023).

A meltdown is often an involuntary and uncontrollable event. When a person is completely overwhelmed, and their condition means that it is difficult to express their feelings in another way, it is understandable that a meltdown may be a consequence. Low adaptive behaviour in combination with greater symptoms of internalising and externalising difficulties may further increase a tendency to meltdown. However, a meltdown is not the only way an autistic person may express feeling overwhelmed; they may also refuse to interact, withdraw from situations they find challenging or avoid situations altogether. Some participants with ASC described what caused them to meltdown or shutdown:

RACHELLE *I guess we can both tell as soon as we start to try and talk to each other what stage I'm at that day ... and we talk about the difference between like a meltdown and a shutdown and sometimes where I'm at the point where I shutdown it's like he doesn't listen straight away when I say it. I have to say it like the third time he listens and that's really frustrating because I'm already at a point where I can't even explain it anymore and I need direction because my brain is not even thinking. It would be nicer if he was a bit more on the ball at those times.*

EDITH *He didn't like me doing a U-turn in the street and parking out the front ... so in his mind he had a model of what we were doing [when parking]. In my mind I was trying to guess ... and then I got it wrong and then he got angry with me ... it was just frustrating and then I did have a meltdown ... He says, 'You never listen', and it's not that I don't listen it's just I don't have the wheels on the cart to listen well and so I got it wrong, and then it was just a simple thing ... I just didn't see what he wanted me to see, and I couldn't understand what he wanted me to do and at every level I was not trying to ignore him but the pattern that I came up with was quite different to the pattern he intended. And I just can't see how I could have done differently.*

Others described what a meltdown or a shutdown was like for them:

WALLY   *Back out, leave the room. No, it doesn't solve the problem, it just allows me to not explode, and I'm not violent or anything, but it's just allows me to not become so emotionally overwhelmed, I just have to extricate myself.*

TOM   *My character is to have calm rational conversations. Sometimes difficult conversations cause me to feel attacked and I respond defensively and sometimes angrily.*

Many people find it hard to tell an autistic meltdown from a temper tantrum because from the outside, they look similar. On the inside, they are a symptom of heightened distress that is undetected, so on the outside the resulting behaviour can look disproportionate to the cause of distress. Behaviours can include emotional outbursts where intense emotions such as anger, frustration, fear or sadness are expressed. These emotions may be amplified and difficult to regulate, leading to intensifying the distress. Although most NT participants indicated that they were trying hard to understand as best they could, still it was difficult for them when they were on the other side of a meltdown:

> WINNIE *It's scary I think, I mean I think at some stages I was actually scared of him … He could be verbally violent. His intensity and as they talk about, the meltdowns, and so forth, I was very scared.*

> SOPHIE *If he is becoming heated towards me, I call him out immediately, strictly and calmly, 'Do not talk to me with that tone' or 'Do not say that to me, it is offensive.' … Often it works for him. If I am the one getting heated, he cannot handle it, in most cases, and has a complete meltdown, with name-calling and tantrum behaviour.*

> HALEY *In the beginning I used to try and reason with him, that was just a waste of time … and I would listen to him … to what he was saying, and he would just get angrier and angrier because I think to him, in his eyes, I wasn't listening to him. That's the way that he has seen it … I don't know, they just keep repeating themselves over and over, 'You*

124

don't understand how I feel.' ... 'Yes, I do understand because you have told me.'... Obviously, a common thread. How do you stop it? ... And neither wins, and the problem is too, that they lose their shit, they are okay straight after it, and you are left suffering for the next week because you are gutted, you are just, you've literally got to scrape yourself off the floor, and then what the f**k just happened? Or even Joe used to always go 'Well you are always so angry at me' and I am thinking 'Well what just happened. Tell me something. Were you in the room? Was I in the same room as you, having this conversation? Am I talking Chinese?'

DAWN   *Going back to your points on the written survey about discussions about things and conversations. We don't. That's another thing where if we are needing to discuss something, let's say our house is on the market, so we were talking about putting our house on the market and we need to discuss something about it ... he gets riled very quickly so we don't really have conversations about things, and he shuts it down ... so the conversation, we each have ... three shots at talking if you like, so 'he says – I say', 'HE SAYS – I SAY', 'HE SAYS – I SAY' and we stop ... and I'm like, okay we will stop at that point because he is getting wound up ... it's not that he is not unhappy with things that I do, obviously because it comes out as a BLAH.*

Have We Gone Nuts?

LUCY   *I don't live with him and never have ... I think*
         I really am lucky because when he starts, I can
         just say, 'Look I've got to go home now', and
         that's the way I've handled it since I found
         out ... That's how I handle that emotional
         hurdle when he starts that, but he doesn't
         communicate ... The only response he's got is
         to find fault in me and blame ... and so it's all
         been very bizarre ... The first eruption I ever
         saw him do is, I took him to a Christmas party
         function where there were about 300 people
         there because it was rather a big company I
         worked for at the time and of course he knew
         no-one and he has this habit of nodding off ...
         everybody had left our table and was mingling
         by then but I just touched him on the knee
         and sort of said, 'You're nodding off'. Well, he
         went for me. 'Don't you tell me what to do,
         don't you!' Growling at me and I said, 'Wow.
         Hang on a minute. You speak to me like that
         I'm out of here and you can catch a cab home'
         ... The verbal. I've never heard him swear like
         it before. He was just off his face. 'You're a this
         and that and that.' I won't repeat it, but ... It
         was bizarre, the first meltdown I'd ever seen
         him have ... and at that point I didn't know
         about Asperger.

A study by Townsend et al. (2022) found another distinctive feature that makes it difficult to distinguish between a meltdown and a temper tantrum. When typical people experience anxiety or distress, they often attempt to avoid what is making them feel anxious or distressed and only tend to engage in problem behaviours after being emotionally provoked. In contrast, Townsend et al. (2022) found that when autistic people experience anxiety, their tendency is to respond immediately to the feared situation with rage attacks or anger outbursts, sometimes to even minor provocations. Often linked to inadequacies in abilities to regulate emotions, ineffective management of overstimulation, or stress, these rage attacks or anger outbursts can exacerbate problems with attention, communication, social interaction and problem-solving abilities (Townsend et al., 2022). Internalising and externalising behaviours can also contribute to intensifying these behaviours.

Whether clinician, counsellor, family member or friend, it is vital to be aware that meltdowns may be a common occurrence in neurodiverse relationships. As each attempt to contend with the resulting fallout of ongoing meltdowns in their own way, various unconventional relational patterns may result. These patterns may include avoidance of speaking about subjects that can set off a meltdown, even if important; appeasing situations by avoidance of certain foods, textures, smells, etc., even if they are the other's preferences; or taking on a heavier workload than previously arranged to keep the peace, just to name a few.

When these behaviours become common, the relationship is at risk of deteriorating. However, the relational patterns that can form as a result of ongoing meltdowns may become the norm in these relationships.

Matters of Maltreatment

Sometimes rage attacks or anger outbursts can result in the mistreatment of others. While abusive behaviour can occur in any individual, regardless of whether they are autistic or not, and abusiveness is not an inherent characteristic of autism, abusive behaviour can arise due to various factors such as personal history, environmental influences, and unaddressed needs or frustrations. It is incorrect and unfair to assume that meltdowns in autistic adults always lead to abusive behaviour. However, autistic adults, like anyone else, can exhibit abusive behaviours if they have not learnt, or been taught, appropriate coping mechanisms, or how to improve communication skills, or emotional regulation techniques. Their propensity to descend into anger rumination also has the potential to escalate into angry outbursts since it depletes abilities to self-regulate and leads to reduced impulse control, hostility or outward expressions of anger. These difficulties can contribute to challenging behaviours, including aggression, yelling or physical harm towards others. Many NT participants described their ASC partner's inability to self-regulate when irritated with them, often over small matters, but this irritation often led to full-blown rage and meltdown. Katy shared how verbal aggression was a regular occurrence in her relationship:

> Gets very aggressive verbally. I don't have any fears about him physically, but verbally he gets very aggressive, very loud, and that is fairly frequent ... He invalidates me all the time and if I didn't have good self-esteem and I wasn't successful in my work life, I'd be a very shattered person.

A Toxic Tailspin

Likewise, Dawn described what took place in heated discussions:

I don't often give vent to my anger, I have internalised, I have held it inside a lot, whilst I noticed when in heated discussion, or when we were in a discussion, he would, if he is in an argument with anybody else, he will win the argument, he is very, very, very good at arguing (sigh). When he is in an argument with me, he loses the plot really quickly. He loses his temper like that and can't handle it. He doesn't become abusive or anything like that, he just boils over very quickly, and I have always observed that. It's like, that's weird why I can stay in control, and for me it's a heated discussion, he has lost the plot, he's just raging, and so angry, that's weird because he doesn't get like that with anybody else.

Diana disclosed that her husband had been physically violent, while also lacking the understanding of the consequences of his behaviour:

I guess a lot of the time things seem to be quite contradictory. He will be very vocal with 'I love you', saying things like that, but his actions kind of say the opposite sometimes. He has been violent in our relationship. He just gets frustrated and gets worked up to such a degree that he then lashes out and is violent and then he's sorry and remorseful and whatever else afterward but he doesn't seem to completely understand that that's not a sign of affection and that he's saying he loves me but then that sort of thing is happening, so yeah, it's just I suppose for him, he doesn't seem to, he can't seem to wrap his head around it.

Then she added that they were both receiving help to overcome this problem:

He is a lot better now than he used to be, we have got on to a very good psychologist, we both see her. She's helping him with his anger management and has been doing that primarily for most of the time he's been seeing her and then recently we've had some joint sessions which have been good to help try and sort through a few issues and problems that have pretty much been there for our whole marriage. We've been married coming up three years and then I see her as well because I mean at least for quite some time I didn't have anyone professionally to see to get help and so that's really helped me to just in general coming to terms with it and even practical help and suggestions, yeah just everyday living, really that's a struggle.

Abuse can unfortunately occur in any type of relationship, including neurodiverse relationships. Abuse in neurodiverse relationships can take various forms, including physical, emotional, verbal, sexual or financial. Although it is also crucial to recognise that these behaviours may be the result of unmet needs, overwhelming sensory experiences, communication difficulties or emotional distress, rather than being intentionally abusive, sometimes, like everyone, abusive behaviour can become intentional. An anonymous survey respondent (NT) said that occurred in her relationship:

When I began to insist on a resolution to important issues, he became dangerous. The level of abuse never abated once it began, but stepped up each time we had a failure of communication, as if some line in the sand kept moving. This led to divorce as the only safe option.

A Toxic Tailspin

It is important to recognise that abuse is never acceptable or justified, regardless of neurodiversity or any other factors. Abuse is a power dynamic where one person seeks to control and dominate the other through harmful actions or behaviours. There are several factors that may contribute to the occurrence of abuse in a neurodiverse relationship:

Communication challenges: Difficulties in communication can lead to misunderstandings, frustration and the potential for conflict. Communication gaps can be exploited by an abusive partner to manipulate or control the other person.

Vulnerability and dependency: Challenges faced in daily living, social interactions or decision-making can create power imbalances in a relationship. An abusive partner may take advantage of resulting vulnerabilities and exert control over the other person.

Lack of support and resources: Limited access to support networks, community resources or appropriate services that can help people recognise and address abusive behaviours. This can also make it more difficult to leave an abusive relationship or seek help.

Stereotypes and stigma: Societal misconceptions and stereotypes can exacerbate power imbalances and contribute to the perpetuation of abusive behaviours. These stereotypes may undermine the experiences and needs of people in neurodiverse relationships, making it harder for them to recognise or disclose abuse.

While abuse is never acceptable, and everyone deserves to be treated with respect, dignity and kindness in their relationships, it is important to understand and recognise reasons behind a potential for abuse to form in a neurodiverse relationship. Diana (NT) illustrated some of these challenges:

With him having this ADD as well … I mean to remember things; he generally always has to ask me. He can't retain a great deal, and even with the psychologist with this anger management … she's had to drill him, because it's taken a long while to get in, and I mean he can still work, and he's handy with his hands, and to a lot of people, he can function fine, and there's not really a problem … The more you're with him it does kind of become obvious that there's something not 100% right. It's really tricky. Often what'll happen is he'll blow up and then you've got to leave it or you've got to come back another time or [if] you still have to deal with it there … because there's no other time to deal with it, it often doesn't end wonderfully well but …. especially with the psychologist we're seeing, time out is the general kind of thing to try and initiate, and she says, 'You've still got to come back to deal with it', so essentially, I guess it does need dealing with, but if he's calmed down. I see a lot of the problem is, he gets angry without realising, or being aware. That's the main problem, and often I've found that it's not even angry necessarily with me. I think a lot of the time he's angry with himself, and he's frustrated, if he can't find words to describe things or whatever it might be. If he's feeling he should be able to do something and can't and then that's when he'll take it out on me, because it's easier to do that and blame, rather than for him to take the responsibility.

While it is important to look out for signs of abusive behaviours in a neurodiverse relationship, it is also important to understand that, although abusive behaviour may be present, the reasons for it may be very different to those of conventional relationships.

Regulating by Rules

Differences to that of a conventional relationship may also appear in a need for adults with ASC to regulate by rules. Since relationships are fluid, they are often unpredictable and messy and are constantly changing as life changes. However, given that people with ASC experience difficulties with social communication together with an intolerance of uncertainty (Rodgers et al., 2018), they often rely on rules and structures to understand and navigate social situations (Robic et al., 2015).

These rules can be self-imposed, or societal norms, that help provide guidance and clarity in social interactions. Deviating from imposed rules, once established, can cause anxiety and confusion. Rigidly keeping everything meticulous, exact and controlled often removes anxiety for those with ASC (Attwood et al., 2014; Petrolini et al., 2023). Therefore, to keep anxiety at bay, rules can be rigidly maintained, and change resisted, even if the rules imposed on others may include adverse consequences for them. This rigidity can extend to various aspects of life, including household rules, routines and expectations held for others. Although Malcolm (ASC) revealed how he wanted things done his way, he also recognised that he could not get his way all the time:

Ah, well I want to give instructions to make things better. I like systems. If I give direction, just do it, it's like system. Like the kids, I will say 'Issy, bring your lunch box in. Take your shoes off ... Issy, just do these things and then you won't have to do them. It is over and done with', or 'Jake, can you go and clean your room before you watch TV.' He will go and watch TV. 'Jake, did you go and do you room?' 'Ahhh!' Ha, ha, ha. I suppose it is frustrating because if it was me, which of course it is, that I am talking about, like planet Malcom, I do it. You do that system ... So, and if people don't do that, I mean I am learning too, to deal with that, obviously, and especially in such a multi-function household as us. I realise that people do things differently. And we will talk about it ... and, yeah, normally either they do it, or they don't. I just back down.

While implementing rules can provide a sense of stability and familiarity in an otherwise unpredictable world, it can present challenges when it comes to adapting to new circumstances or being open to different perspectives. When rigidly insisting on a set of rules to maintain a need for sameness and predictability within a relationship, it can lend itself to narrow ideas about the way in which life should happen. While making and keeping rules is to feel safe, it can be a struggle to understand a different impact of the rules on others. Fiona (NT) shared that she was mainly confined to doing what William (ASC) wanted:

Mainly William's stubbornness confines me into what he wants done, so therefore as a partnership, we can't do what we both want, so therefore stubbornness is a tool to basically get your own way.

It is important for both autistic and neurotypical individuals to find a balance between maintaining stability and embracing necessary changes. Patience, understanding and clear communication can help navigate these situations. However, if compromise is not able to be established, the result can be the proliferation of rigid inflexibility. Strongly held opinions combined with an all or nothing type of thinking may cause compromise to be viewed negatively. When there is a perception that opinions and preferences are either right or wrong, finding a grey area may feel like 'losing'. In that instance, finding common ground with another's point of view may become almost impossible. It may also be a reason that abusive behaviour develops. Beth (NT) described how needing to be right kept Christopher (ASC) finding fault with her:

> *He's always got to be right. Always, yeah and everything is always my fault. Yeah, everything is, well everyone else's fault except theirs, and he corrects my grammar. And I get really cranky … because if he thinks he's right, and he's wrong he won't have it … so it sort of just comes to a stalemate.*

Katy (NT) shared how compromise did not appear to be in Ronald's (ASC) vocabulary:

> *If he doesn't want to do something he just doesn't do it. You cannot force him to do anything he doesn't want to do, and I mean this is one of the lonely spots in our relationship, is that he will be motivated to do something that he wants to do but for me to ask him to do something, it's like I have asked him to pin himself to a cross. It is just so resistive, and he might do it eventually, after months and months of me asking, but he will do it with such foul temper that it is almost a waste of me getting anything done. And it never gets finished. He never finishes anything that he doesn't want to do.*

However, since NT people have the ability to take perspective, which means that they can imagine the thoughts and feelings behind requests, it is more likely that they may accommodate others. When negotiating with others, they usually have a greater capacity to be flexible with the give and take required to 'meet halfway' and to make necessary adjustments. In a neurodiverse relationship, a desire to please and promote unity may become a pattern of deferring to the wishes of the person with autism, just to keep the peace. Sometimes this behaviour may become the status quo of a relationship. Ryan (NT) shared how this was often the case in his relationship:

Usually, you have two people and people with two different agendas and in a partnership, you usually amalgamate that agenda to an agreed upon agenda to work off. She is not very good at that; compromise and negotiation are not things she thinks to involve herself with. She doesn't understand why what 'she wants' shouldn't be what 'we want'. And we often struggle, and for her ... to say something is to do it, whereas with me, I am quite strong in neurotypical in a lot of ways, for me, I mull things over, I think about things, I look at other aspects to it. Even I might sit on it before coming to a decision about something, but she makes a decision quite quickly and acts on it, so you know if I say 'Oh, thinking about going to a conference on the weekend', she will automatically go and book my accommodation, transport for it. It's her way of being nice to me and showing love and support for me, but it may not have actually been a case that I actually wanted to go to it. I am expressing a liking or longing to go to it, but not a need, not something I would actually go and do. She has trouble understanding the difference between people putting out ideas of flying kites and floating ideas ... If there is peace to be made, I am mostly the person that makes the peace and so if there is an apology to be given, even if it is not my fault, I will apologise just to keep things on an even keel, and some of that was explained to Rachelle to how other relationships work.

Similarly, Laura (NT) shared how she accommodated her ASC partner:

On daily basis warm tone of voice, calm voice, smiles, questions regarding wishes or feelings, and a great deal of practical doing and caring activity – meals, changing household routines to meet his exacting cleanliness standards, to meet his erratic schedule and eating phobias. Changing household lighting at his 'indirect' request. Endless compromise about household routine – how dishes are washed, how food is prepared. Adjustment to his night owl schedule.

Considering that instigating rules helps create a framework for a person on the spectrum to feel safe and more in control of the environment, enforcing 'the right way of doing things' is a way for those on the spectrum to ensure that the largely confusing aspect of relating is somewhat less confusing (Petrolini et al., 2023). However, there cannot be a rule for every eventuality and rules cannot be unequivocally followed all the time. In addition, others tend to push back on rules and preferences imposed on them, which may cause a person on the spectrum to become emotionally dysregulated or feel overwhelmed, have difficulties controlling impulsive behaviours or have angry outbursts. Meltdowns, shutdowns, or in some cases, abusive behaviour may then follow.

Managing by Mandates

Another potential nonconformity to that of a conventional relationship may result from the autistic need to rigidly control their environment (Petrolini et al., 2023) and therefore control others in their relationships. Controlling behaviour can occur in any individual, regardless of whether they are autistic or not. However, the motives may be different. A strong need for control can stem from a desire for predictability, as unexpected changes can be overwhelming and anxiety-inducing. Establishing routines and predictability can help autistic people navigate the world more comfortably. In relationships, this need for control may manifest in many different ways. They may want to impose their own set of rules or expectations on others for how interactions should unfold. They may prefer to plan and structure activities or have specific expectations for how things should be done. They may struggle with relinquishing control or sharing control in certain situations to safeguard consistency. Often, they do not intend to be tyrannical, but are highly overwhelmed by the world around them. William (ASC) indicated that his need to try to keep tight control on his reactions was a response to an inability to respond.

I have to overcome a fear barrier to do anything ... and add on top of that Asperger's, which is a natural proclivity anyway. It's a wonder I can function at all ... Your brain is a chemical thing, physical. It may feel in certain ways, but you don't have to ... because we do have control. Most people are subject to their brains' chemistry, and of course, it's a spontaneous thing, and what probably makes normal NT behaviour what it is. Respond instantly to emotional responses. Create them from recognising in others. I can't do that so at least I can keep on an even keel by controlling, keeping a tight control. Otherwise, you're going up and down without knowing why.

If, on the other hand, a neurodiverse relationship has spiralled into severe disenchantment, or into complete rigid inflexibility, it can begin to feel like a dictatorship. When an adult with ASC meets ongoing resistance to their need for rigidity, they may form an adversarial view of their NT partner or family member. People on the autism spectrum are naturally self-focused, and mindblindness does not enable them to easily put context toward many of the expectations held by others. If others begin to be viewed by an autistic adult as an encumbrance to their own peace and pleasure in life, they may be considered as an adversary, or a rival to getting their own needs met. This type of thinking may result in the formation of coercive control, which is a pattern of controlling and manipulative behaviours to provoke particular responses within a relationship (Stark & Hester, 2018). Haley (NT) described how control had begun to dominate her relationship:

He never listens to me anyway, maybe in the beginning, but as our marriage went on, he just liked to be in control, and if you take the control away, then he finds it very hard to deal with … I just think that it was more we did things just to make him happy … it was just easier to do things that he wanted to do or to do it his way … like we went to Sydney for our 10th wedding anniversary and … he has nothing planned to that evening. We just got there, and I go, 'Oh wow! Sydney, we haven't been here for years!' So I wanted to go and have a look and walk around and I got abused you know. 'We've got the same f**king shops in Brisbane.

What do you want to go look at them here for?' I thought, 'Whoa okay.' So, then we rushed back up to the motel and sat there and did nothing, watched TV. I wasn't allowed to walk around and have a look and it was the same thing over the weekend. We had this helicopter ride booked as my surprise, which was lovely. Once again, and I'll give him his due, probably the biggest thing he had ever planned on his own for me, but the thing was he loves helicopters, not me. He did what he wanted to do and I'm happy to shop, I love walking and he doesn't like walking ... and I was just so upset because all I wanted to do then was to walk around the Botanical Gardens which we were across the road. Oh, couldn't do that! Oh, it was just nothing! Yes, so that's probably a prime example.

Likewise, Nora (NT) described some of her partner's controlling ways:

Some things that I tell him, he's just like 'Nah you're not going to tell me what to do'... He naturally is resistant to cooperating. He even says it himself ... 'I just like to buck. I don't want to do what everybody else is doing. I just like to buck against everything.' He's a rogue but somehow, I've managed to tame him, in some regards.

On the other hand, Ryan (NT) described how Rachelle (ASC) controlled the environment and crossed boundaries to make herself comfortable:

She is also the kind of person that will walk in somewhere and have an attitude of taking, not taking control, but you know the familiar, like ... she will go in somewhere and she will change a radio station to what she likes to listen to rather than what the person likes to listen to, but ... God forbid they do that to her! Or she will put her feet up on the table or something like that. She will do stuff that, it crosses a boundary, a social boundary of what you are allowed to get away with, with that degree of familiarity with a person. She doesn't understand that there's a graduated boundary, the more you know someone the more you can do.

Although Winnie (NT) understood that her ASC partner may be experiencing anxiety or struggles, his need to control engulfed her:

I must admit I am not as logical sequential organised as he is, and so we are at great odds in how we approach things, so his level of frustration is easily tipped over. And he also finds that in his work as well, that if somebody speaks to him and rambles then he will just want to hang up on them. He said, 'You are not telling me, tell me the message ... I can't work it out', and so it is that sort of structured world, so if the domestic world isn't structured the way that he wants it or the work world doesn't present in a comprehensible way, he will have high levels of frustration ... Those sorts of issues on the domestic scene would have caused a fight, but now I have to 'bite my tongue' or just accept that it's ... not his need to be right, it is more about his anxiety, [his] need to control it by things being a certain way ... It is normally an indicator to me that he is struggling with something in the work environment so he brings it home and that is how it will be ... expressed. He won't say 'I've had a bad day at work', he will go in and he will nitpick everything I do.

When relationships sink into an oppositional dynamic, the cumulative effect of accommodating a person's needs at the expense of one's own needs, while also needing to be alert to the moment a meltdown or shutdown may be imminent, can create a sense of hypervigilance. This may give rise to a sense of danger, which can instil fear and result in outward expressions of anger. Laura (NT) revealed how she often had to censor herself:

I have to watch my emotions and tongue so as not to wound him or present him with stuff that upsets him.

Fiona (NT) described the anger she felt due to William's (ASC) oppositional ways:

I don't have the energy to put in for reinventing the wheel every day, so then we just become less patient, then every day becomes another day, another bloody argument. I don't want to live like that. Yeah, so it's not a happy situation. It is not happy for him. It's not happy for me. But I don't, I really don't see the solution ... So you've got this person on this side thinking you're a crazy bitch, because the way you're behaving ... So it is a bit difficult to get things done because he just says to me 'Don't tell me what to do. End of story!' I walk away ... It's not going to work because he is taking my words up the wrong way. So I am better off just being quiet. Going and doing it myself. I try to explain to him, then it comes down to 'I'm not explaining it in the words that he wants', and then it usually escalates into an argument. So once again another day, another argument. So it's not working at the moment ... Draining and frustrating. And sometimes I just say 'You drive me crazy. Absolutely crazy'. I used to yell it at him. Now I just say it. Because it is not helping my health to get so het up about it. I'm trying to change the way I interact with him, but what I'm finding is not changing because he is bringing in new behaviours that keeps us in that conflict situation. And that's why I hope someone can get through to him because I can't. Can't, and I don't want to stay in that conflict. I want to move on. Life's too short.

Whereas William conveyed that although he had observed many instances of Fiona's expressions of anger, he did not understand what caused it or what to do about it:

It really seems that NTs are really pre-programmed in a whole lot of ways and if they don't get the reactions they expect, it brings up an emotional response. It's most unfortunate. And that's this anger problem that we can't understand. And I've read a lot of entries from people writing on the internet forums. It's one of the topics that [I] cannot understand, these reactions ... all we can do is to be quite neutral, and even that causes anger. What can you do? You can't do anything.

Increasingly, research is finding that many NT partners and family members in neurodiverse relationships experience chronic stress (Arad et al., 2022; Millar-Powell & Warburton, 2020; Rench, 2014). Chronic stress often results from being governed by rules or dominated by control in a relationship. According to Russell and Lightman (2019) chronic stress leads to long-term cortisol exposure 'which can lead to a broad range of problems including the metabolic syndrome, obesity, cancer, mental health disorders, cardiovascular disease and increased susceptibility to infections' (p. 525).

In the interest of health and wellbeing, for all concerned, it is essential to correct the imbalances that frequently occur in neurodiverse relationships. Furthering our understanding of the roles and interactions between the different cognitive mechanisms, the internalising or externalising difficulties those with ASC experience and their need to implement rules and controlling strategies to compensate is important for developing better understanding and more effective and targeted interventions (Ozsivadjian et al., 2021).

Support Thoughts

Usually, a person on the spectrum does not intend to be dictatorial. They are often highly overwhelmed by the world around them, and making rules and keeping tight control on their environment helps them feel safe. Consequently, they struggle to understand the impact of their rules and controls on those around them. They also often report that they feel that it is unfair to have to learn a lot of strategies to make NT people feel happy, when they are only trying to make themselves happy.

Whether clinician, counsellor, family member or friend, it can be helpful to expand their theory of mind by examining ways in which the NT people in their lives have been accommodating their autistic brain throughout their time together. They may be quite surprised to think about all the ways their NT loved ones have silently shown love by keeping the needs of their ASC partners and family members ever-present in their minds for the entirety of their life together.

Sometimes a person on the spectrum has genuinely thought that their loved ones prefer silent meals, enjoys the same food, or likes the same things without realising that they are being accommodated to keep the family home peaceful and functional. With assistance, people with ASC may be motivated to learn that the mood, energy levels and attitudes toward them might greatly improve if there was effort on their part to build the skills necessary to improve reciprocity in the relationship. While these aspects may seem obvious to NT people, cause and effect is sometimes quite challenging for the ASC brain and abstract concepts like reciprocity and mutuality need to be broken down into specifics. There is always hope for a relationship when all concerned are willing to learn, bend and grow.

The next chapter focuses on how the differences between NT and ASC people may cause a needs deprivation between them.

6

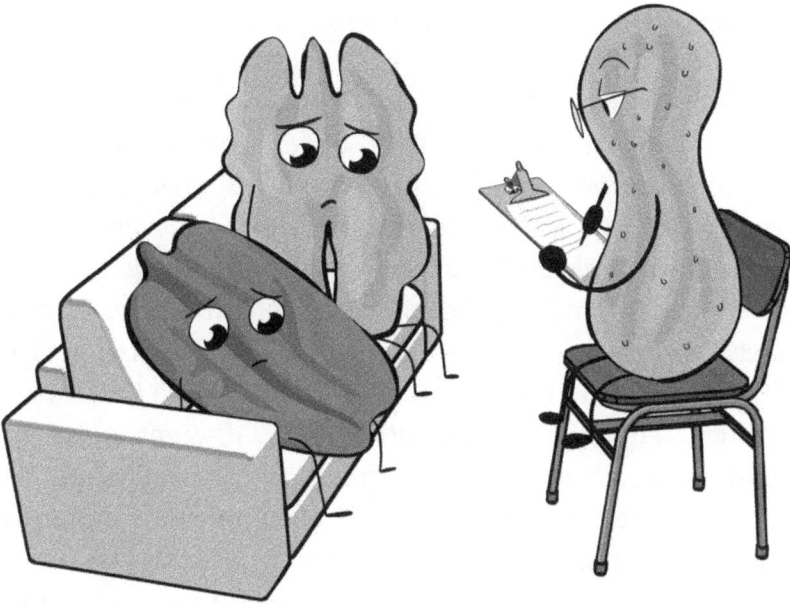

Needs Deprivation

Have We Gone Nuts?

'We're only as needy as our unmet needs.'
John Bowlby

The many differences between NT and ASC people discussed so far and the subsequent difficulties that occur between them when they are in a relationship together, may result in a needs deprivation for each. The lack of understanding and awareness of each other's neurological differences (Huggins et al., 2021) can make it difficult to recognise and address each other's needs, potentially leading to emotional disconnection and deprivation. The communication differences that result in a communication gap (Kushki et al., 2021) can bring about unmet needs and a lack of understanding. The sensory sensitivities that many autistic adults experience (Hwang et al., 2020) can affect their ability to meet their own needs or be receptive to the needs of others. The cognitive functioning challenges those with autism experience (Berenguer et al., 2018; Powell et al., 2017) may mean they struggle to meet their own needs or support others effectively, leading to feelings of a needs deprivation on both sides. The differences in tolerances for unpredictability and abilities to adapt to the resulting ups and downs of life (Petrolini et al., 2023), potentially leads to emotional disconnection and a needs deprivation on both sides. The commonly accepted social expectations and norms that are challenging to navigate for many autistic people (Arioli et al., 2018; Hull et al., 2017) can contribute to feelings of isolation, a lack of fulfillment, tension and unmet needs for both.

While a significant needs divergence contributes, in part, to the unconventional features of neurodiverse relationships, so too does the way in which each attempt to get their individual

148

needs met. The ASC desire to avoid interpersonal interaction, as opposed to the NT desire to engage in interpersonal interaction reported in Book 1 causes an impasse in abilities for each to get their needs met. This impasse, together with the degree of difference between the two types of people in neurodiverse relationships means that there is a high probability that most people in these relationships will experience a needs deprivation in differing degrees.

Different proficiencies in empathy or mentalising (Fitzgerald, 2020; Rueda et al., 2015), different motivations to be connected with others (Lockwood et al., 2017) and different perceptions and expectations of close relationships (Finke, 2023; Heasman & Gillespie, 2017) are additional contrasts between ASC and NT people that may also intensify a needs deprivation in these relationships.

Empathy Has Many Faces

Empathy is the ability to understand and share the feelings, emotions and perspectives of others and is considered an essential aspect of social cognition (Lockwood et al., 2017). Thought to be similar to mentalising (also referred to as theory of mind), both are psychological concepts that involve understanding and relating to the mental states of others. Therefore, both empathy and ToM involve the ability to understand and appreciate the thoughts, feelings and perspectives of others. Both concepts allow people to mentally simulate and comprehend what someone else might be experiencing. Both concepts can be described as the ability to share others' feelings or to be able to 'put yourself in their shoes', imagining what they might be experiencing, and relating to their emotions. Both concepts are crucial for effective social interactions. They enable people to navigate social situations, form social bonds and engage in prosocial behaviour.

Although empathy and ToM are similar, both concepts have distinct characteristics that are interconnected and contribute to our overall social understanding and interactions. While both play essential roles in our ability to relate to others, they emphasise different aspects of social cognition and understanding. It's important to note that empathy is distinct from sympathy. While empathy involves understanding and sharing emotions, sympathy refers to feeling pity or compassion for someone without necessarily experiencing their emotions. Empathy allows you to connect with others on a deeper level. It plays a crucial role in building and maintaining healthy relationships. It helps foster trust, understanding and effective communication. It enables people to offer compassion, support and assistance to those in need, as they can better grasp the challenges and emotions faced by others.

It has been thought that autistic people did not experience empathy. It is now known that empathy exists on a spectrum in people with ASC, just as it does in NT people. However, due to differences in neurology, individuals with ASC often have unique patterns of empathy. Some may experience challenges in recognising and understanding others' emotions and perspectives, which can affect their ability to respond empathetically. However, this does not mean individuals with ASC lack empathy entirely. They may demonstrate empathy in different ways or have difficulty expressing it in conventional ways.

Needs Deprivation

Empathy is a complex cognitive and emotional process which can manifest differently in different people, regardless of neurodiversity. It is a multi-dimensional concept which includes cognitive empathy, affective empathy, state empathy and trait empathy (McKenzie et al., 2021). Cognitive empathy refers to the ability to understand and take the perspective of others. It involves recognising and comprehending the thoughts, beliefs, intentions and emotions of others (Rueda et al., 2015). Cognitive empathy and mentalising are sometimes considered interchangeable, but there are mounting evidence to suggest that these constructs have different underlying neurobiological mechanisms (Clutterbuck et al., 2021). This aspect of empathy allows people to intellectually understand what others might be experiencing without necessarily sharing the same emotional response. In autism, cognitive empathy can be impaired to varying degrees, with autistic people often struggling to interpret social cues, understand others' emotions, or predict others' behaviours based on nonverbal cues.

Affective empathy is the emotional response from one to another (Smith, 2009). It is also known as emotional empathy or empathy driven by emotions, which involves sharing and experiencing the emotions of others. It refers to the capacity to emotionally resonate with another person's feelings and respond with appropriate emotions. People high in affective empathy can automatically and instinctively feel what others are feeling. In autism, affective empathy can also be impaired, with autistic people having difficulties in spontaneously sharing or understanding others' emotional experiences.

Empathic accuracy refers to the ability to accurately identify and understand the emotional states and thoughts of others (McKenzie et al., 2021). It involves accurately perceiving and interpreting both verbal and nonverbal emotional cues, which enables people to respond appropriately. Empathic accuracy goes beyond cognitive and affective empathy by emphasising the accuracy of empathic responses. In the context of autism, empathic accuracy can be challenging, as individuals may struggle to accurately perceive and interpret social cues, leading to difficulties in accurately understanding and responding to others' emotional states.

Empathy can be further divided into trait empathy and state empathy (Song et al., 2019). State empathy is context dependent; namely, it is a short-term instant psychological state in response to a specific stimulus or situation. In contrast, trait empathy is relatively stable across time and different situations. It does not require a specific situation or stimulus, but instead is a person's overall tendency to be able to understand and share the emotions and feelings of other people (Song et al., 2019). Therefore, although it is well known that empathy is a key element in the ability to connect with and understand others (Ciaunica, 2019), there is a complexity to it that is still not yet fully understood.

That said, it is important to note that people with autism can have a wide range of empathic abilities, and not all people with autism will experience impairments in all aspects of empathy. Some people with autism may demonstrate strengths in specific areas of empathy, while others may experience challenges across multiple dimensions. The degree of impairment or strength in empathy can vary from person to person, highlighting the heterogeneity of the autism condition. Wally (ASC) described how empathy functioned for him:

I wish I could find a way to express an empathic response without becoming overwhelmed … I read all the stuff about the four domains of empathy. I know where I fit within that. I know that personal distress thing, there it is – bang! So, I wish I could actually do the mirroring and I wish I could truly say, 'I understand how you feel' in a way that anyone else can accept, rather than becoming overwhelmed and in need of support myself. That's the thing; I can't. If somebody needs support … within that exchange if the person that I'm with needs emotional support, ultimately, it's me that needs the support … I sit there on the other side to a student who is in tears … and trying to figure out what's going on and I can sit there, and I can talk them through their options and … I can help them feel better and then I need to go for a long walk. But in where I'm already invested in it, no!

Although the experience of empathy can vary widely, many NT participants described the ASC people in their lives as lacking empathy:

DANA   *I find that there is a lot of work on my part to manage the relationship. My son tends to really lack empathy, so you may say to him for example, 'I've had this cold, Jay. I'm sick' … and he goes, 'Oh well, you know when you have a cold, what to do, just go drink water'… I expect a little bit more loving care, the way I give to him, and I never ever get it, so I've learned to just not expect that thing from him … he'll be 30 in December, and I remember when he was a small child, he was extremely loving … Trying to just kind of remind him about empathy. He will tell you*

*that he does not have empathy. He will tell
you that he should not have empathy because
he is a warrior. He believes he is a warrior …
and he thinks that empathy would make him
weak or at least this is how he rationalises it in
his mind … I didn't really understand about
what Asperger's did to adults … the kind of
empathy thing that he was not getting. He
estranged from me for a year and then … a
year later I get this text, 'Well I'm ready to
talk, if you're ready to talk'. I'm like, 'Okay,
I'd like to talk too' … Oh my gosh, if I could
only just get him to catch that little glimmer
of what other people are feeling.*

GEORGIA   *Do they have that capacity for compassion in
that way or can they genuinely only feel for
themselves? I mean my husband recognises
that I get anxious. I think he knows what
anxiety feels like because he's experienced
that himself but to be able to be compassionate
towards me when I'm anxious, I've not
experienced that in the way that I feel I
would like to experience it; in the way that I
get that from my friends. If I'm anxious and
I express that I'm anxious, they reciprocate
with reassurances and all the other appropriate
behaviours and responses, but with him, if
I were to express, 'I'm anxious', then it's,
'You're overreacting', or he will make it sort
of logic as to why I should not be feeling that
way, which is I guess that speaks of their logic
way of thinking and just intellectualising.*

Needs Deprivation

RYAN   *I feel that she does enough in a sense to try to satisfy my needs emotionally. She certainly tries. I do give her some leeway knowing that she does have an issue in terms of empathy around the whole ASD stuff, but what she wants from me in return, it doesn't sort of align with what her idea is of that. Like she expects a lot more contact, phone calls, token gifts and things like that … but I don't know whether it's a real internal need for her to have that or it's a need she thinks has to be fulfilled because that's how it works in couples, or what she has observed because a lot of what she does is kind of cognitive reasoning around how things should work instead of having intuitive knowledge of how things work. Hard for me to describe, she has to kind of write things out, think things out, and try and work out … what a neurotypical would probably just automatically intuitively understand and do or expect.*

Even though empathy is often thought to be an automatic response, recent theories have argued that motivation plays a key role in modulating empathic experiences (Lockwood et al., 2017). In other words, empathy is felt for others when people are motivated to empathise with them, but not so much when lacking this motivation. Lacking the motivation to be empathetic with others can be influenced by various factors and is not exclusive to individuals with autism. It's important to recognise that empathy requires effort and emotional investment, and there can be several reasons why someone may struggle with motivation in this regard. Some potential factors could include:

Emotional overload: Some people may find it challenging to empathise with others due to their own emotional struggles or being overwhelmed by their own emotions. This can make it difficult to extend empathy towards others.

Personal experiences: Past negative experiences, trauma or personal difficulties may make it harder for someone to connect with and empathise with others. It can lead to emotional distancing as a coping mechanism.

Lack of understanding: Empathy requires understanding and perspective-taking. If someone lacks knowledge or awareness about different experiences or struggles, they may find it challenging to empathise with others.

Emotional detachment: Some people may have a tendency towards emotional detachment or have difficulties in connecting with their own emotions. This can make it more challenging for them to connect with and understand the emotions of others.

Lack of social skills: Empathy is closely linked to social skills and emotional intelligence. If someone has deficits in these areas, they may struggle to demonstrate empathy towards others.

To fully support people in neurodiverse relationships, it is essential to realise that experiences of empathetic responses in their relationships will often be quite different to what is believed usual for close relationships. Without this understanding, it may be difficult to appreciate the specific complications that may result and consequently be unable to develop appropriately targeted supports and interventions, both for those with autism and their partners and family members.

A Question of Disinclination

While motivation appears to be an influence on empathic experiences for most people, motivation may also play a role in the inclination to connect with others, particularly for those on the spectrum. Social connectedness is defined as a sense of belonging and the psychological bond that people have with others (Haslam et al., 2015). It results from a desire and motivation to engage in social interactions and form relationships with others. It is well known that people with ASC have less desire and less motivation to connect socially with others in comparison to NT people. In other words, rather than the typical tendencies toward emotional connection that most people expect, people on the spectrum often display a disinclination to connect.

To understand this disinclination, León (2019) puts forward the idea that those with ASC experience impairments in the capacity to connect with the feelings and actions of others because of a lack of involvement in social reciprocity. This lack of involvement means that people on the spectrum need to rely on intellectual and cognitive strategies to learn about the social world, however, these strategies are insensitive to the moment-by-moment changes of real-life social interactions. Relying on such strategies makes it difficult to reciprocate with others in meaningful ways, and often, the process may be avoided altogether – it then can become almost impossible to learn how to engage in the process of reciprocity.

Adding to this notion, Koldewyn et al. (2013) introduces the idea that a lack of involvement may be more about disinterest than disability. They state that 'people with ASD show a disinclination, not a disability, in global processing, and highlight the broader question of whether other characteristics of autism may also reflect disinclinations rather than disabilities' (p. 2329). In their study, Koldewyn et al. (2013) found that, when explicitly instructed, people with ASC can display abilities in some areas where they usually exhibit inabilities. In some instances, this can indicate a disinclination rather than disability. The question remains regarding motivation. Does a lack of motivation lead to the inability or does an inability lead to a lack of motivation?

A similar disinclination was found in my studies. As reported in Book 1, people with ASC could interact socially when prompted to do so. However, they discontinued social interaction when not prompted. For example, Ruth (NT) found that connection with her partner was possible if she kept prompting with questions:

With prompting, my husband tries to put forth the effort to connect with me, not just share information. I am the one who has to ask him questions in an effort to connect. He doesn't go out of his way to connect with me … I wish I didn't have to prompt him … but I realise that is the reality of my life … He needs instructions, so if I provide them, he can usually follow them in his own way … It would be great if he could say these things without prompting, but I know that may never happen.

While, in the main, the inclination to be connected with others can be quite different between ASC and NT people, it is important to recognise that individuals with autism are a diverse group, and not all autistic individuals will have the same experiences or preferences. However, many ASC and NT participants confirmed these differences. The ASC group described how they were contented with less connection than their NT partners and family members:

> SHARON   *In my previous marriage to my NT partner, I have found that our expectations and requirements for emotional connection were quite different. I was craving more personal space and time while he was wanting to do many things together.*

> TOM   *I feel comfortable when I am with Ken and I do not feel lonely. To me that is a satisfactory emotional connection. I don't know how to make warm affectionate conversations, but I don't feel anything lacking. Sometimes [he] says our intimacy is lacking.*

In contrast to the ASC group, most NT participants showed substantial dissatisfaction to this state of affairs:

> NORA   *Well obviously we've both got different emotional needs ... and basically there's a disparity there which means I'm lumped with how it is ... and when I say to him are you happy, he goes, 'Yeah, I've got no problems with you. This is great for me, this relationship.' I'm like, 'I'm glad you're so happy.'*

Have We Gone Nuts?

SABRINA   I'm the one who's dissatisfied. He's kind of okay because he's getting whatever limited needs that he has met.

Some potential factors that may inhibit an inclination to be connected with others could include the challenges in social communication and interaction autistic people often face. Some people with autism may have a strong desire for social connection and actively seek social interaction but struggle with the necessary social skills, or face difficulties in interpreting social cues. They may find initiating and maintaining conversations, understanding nonverbal communication or comprehending social norms challenging, which can sometimes lead to feelings of isolation or exclusion.

On the other hand, some autistic people may have a reduced inclination to be connected with others, primarily due to factors such as sensory sensitivities, social anxiety or a preference for solitary activities. They may find social interactions overwhelming or exhausting, and as a result, may choose to limit their social engagements. This does not necessarily mean that they do not value connections or relationships, but rather that their preferences and comfort levels in social situations may differ from neurotypicals.

It's important to note that these differences in the inclination to be connected with others are not exclusive to autism and can also vary among neurotypical people. Not all neurotypical people have the same degree of social connectedness, and some may also have a preference for solitude or experience challenges in social interactions. Understanding and respecting these individual differences is crucial in fostering inclusive and supportive environments that accommodate the needs and preferences of all people, regardless of their neurodiversity.

Preferences, Perceptions and Partnerships

Collaboration is the action of working with someone to produce something. Usually, when people form a relationship, they work collaboratively to build a life together, to obtain a home and to create a family. However, in order to reach the level of collaboration necessary to achieve a healthy, functioning home, it is important to have shared values and goals to create a sense of unity and purpose in a relationship. To do this it is important to be able to discuss and align aspirations, dreams and values to ensure that each person understands the other's perspective so that they may move in a similar direction.

However, due to their diverse neurocognitive profiles and social experiences, relationships between ASC and NT people are usually influenced by each having different perceptions and expectations. A study by Finke (2023) revealed that there is mounting evidence 'to suggest autistic individuals have preferences about how they want to act in their socially significant relationships and that these preferences may differ from the preferences and actions of some (if not many or most) non-autistic people' (p. 3056). Finke (2023) also reports that 'for years autistics have been telling researchers they have a preference for less closeness (both emotional and physical) with their friends' (p. 3057). This autistic preference may not necessarily always bring friendships to an end, as friendships may be able to survive with less closeness; however, it can be a different matter when applied to close relationships. Although there is significant variability within the autism spectrum, usually when in a relationship with an NT individual (someone who commonly wants higher levels of affection and connection) a preference for less closeness may become a source of heartache. Dana (NT) shared the pain of losing contact with her autistic son, while also trying to make sense of what kept him from wanting to reconnect with her:

> *I can say regarding the estrangement issue which has been very, very painful is that in learning about this, I have quite frankly become more accepting of my younger son's choice to estrange from me and everyone else in the family because he's estranged not only from me but … his father, certainly his brother, all of his extended family including his grandparents, cousins, aunts and uncles, doesn't have anything to do with anyone … He doesn't have any way of understanding his impulses and his reactions to other people and he doesn't really know how to come back and now I understand that. I thought he was choosing to reject me, and I couldn't figure out what I did to be rejected, I just didn't know. I was asking him and writing letters and 'Please tell me what I did wrong. I want to work with you. Please I can help you. You need to just talk to me.' … I did everything.*

When asked 'Did he respond to you', she answered *'Nope'*.

An anonymous survey respondent (NT) revealed a similar difficulty:

> *My son is 20 years old and has stopped communicating with me completely. He doesn't look at me and hasn't spoken to me in 18 months. I have no idea what to do. Anyone I've talked to says there's nothing I can do until he decides he's ready to get help.*

Needs Deprivation

Sabrina (NT) shared how an ongoing lack of closeness between her and her partner, meant that eventually she stopped giving attention to her marriage:

I've kind of coped, come up with ways to cope with it, it doesn't bother me so much anymore ... because I know it's just a waste of my time and it's just not going to go anywhere. He just doesn't get it. Even my mum still tries to figure out ways and I'm like, 'Mum you're wasting your time. He just doesn't get it. You've got to accept that he doesn't get it, so it's just a waste of time.' It's really sad. I mean I've really given up on just the whole marriage and try to concentrate my efforts on what I'm going to do going forward.

Similarly, Holly (NT) revealed that she had accepted a lack of closeness in her relationship:

Once I would have pursued at all costs if he walked away or if he seemed to be disinterested. I would have come back to it like a dog with a bone but now we've got the diagnosis I now think just let it go. Just live on the surface because that's all he's capable of. I think going away on the weekend when all us women got together some of them will have answered your survey, we got together for a weekend and when I heard their experiences it was a terrible, terrible disappointment ... but within a short while ... I bobbed back up because it was almost like I thought, 'Okay I've got my answer now. It can't be fixed.' ... I guess I moved from angry to accepting ... I still go back into anger sometimes, but I've got far more accepting and I'm just not looking for it anymore.

Anonymous survey responses revealed different reactions to an ongoing disconnection in their relationships:

163

Have We Gone Nuts?

Rightly or wrongly, I have taken the stance that reasoning with each and every drama of the day is little to do with me. There is little point offering an opinion that is most likely going to be disregarded.

After all these years, I keep trying to keep us connected. My husband needs so little from the emotional side of our relationship. We've gotten through all these years because what I call 'The Corporation' is so very good. We only know now, in the last few years exactly why we can't 'fix' the problems in our relationship. We are both still grieving over that. At times I slip into anger and resentment, and he feels depression and self-loathing. He has finally let me see beyond his self-described 'character role' to learn about how he actually thinks and feels. This complete honesty is what has broken both our hearts and yet given us a new chance at a more meaningful, real relationship.

I have explained to my partner that the way I feel connected to him is through talking and that it is hard for me to maintain a feeling of connectedness when he barely responds. He made more effort for a while but seems to have given up; perhaps it is too hard. I try cognitively to value all the actions he does which show me he cares because he does do lots of nice things for me, but somehow, they don't mean as much to me as a conversation. I have to deliberately think about the things he does and place value on them. There is not the automatic satisfaction that comes with a meaningful conversation.

It's become second nature, now, to avoid emotional responses and getting angry, because I know that my emotion will cause an overload, everything will escalate, and the situation will be dreadful for many days. It's better to remain factual and emotionally neutral. I deliberately don't think a lot about how much emotional warmth I would like in our relationship, because it's not going to happen like it seems to in other couples. Why torment myself? It's better to get on with life and learn how to make it work as best we can.

I have let go of most of my expectations of this relationship. I find it easier to think of him as a friend. Six years on, my mental health is better, and I make me happy. Age helps; I'm 64.

Even in the course of differences and difficulties, the capacity to work together with others can be improved through an ability to accommodate others' perspectives. Perspective taking refers to the ability to understand and consider the perspectives, thoughts and feelings of others. It makes interactions more easily interpretable and provides common ground for continued engagement (Cooke et al., 2018). It plays a crucial role in social interactions and empathetic understanding.

However, autistic people may experience challenges in perspective taking, particularly in social contexts. Since they often find it difficult to infer the thoughts, intentions and mental states of others based on social cues, body language and contextual information, they can misunderstand others' intentions. Relying more heavily on explicit, verbal information rather than implicit cues when trying to understand others' perspectives, their more concrete thinking style can make it harder to grasp the abstract or nuanced mental states of others. This can sometimes result in difficulties in predicting or anticipating the behaviours and reactions of their NT partners and family members. Ruth (NT) shared her frustrations about their different perspectives that led to disharmony between them:

It seems like every time I THINK we are on the same page, I come to find out that we are not ... We will discuss an important matter ... he will agree with me ... on a course of action, and then a few days later he won't follow the plan we had discussed. When he does this, I don't really feel like following it either because I say to myself 'What is the point when he just goes off and does B again instead of what we talked about and agreed to?' It looks rather selfish to me when he does this. His reasons make sense to him, but not to me. I feel unheard and disrespected, and then we do it all over again with the next important conversation.

Rose (NT) agreed with this sentiment:

In conversations I guess the biggest challenge is ... if we're taking it in two different directions and especially if I get frustrated about it because Pierre is already trying really hard ... I feel bad because I know it's not really fair to him and it's just a miscommunication, but I get really frustrated because I do really want to be going from the same page.

Dianne (NT) described how life can get 'weird' due to their different perspectives:

We will go for a walk. We will have brekkie and walk back in the sun and then come home and something will go wrong and so we'll go off and then he will go outside and do his thing. I will do mine and then later in the afternoon he will come and say, 'You want a cup of tea?' and we will sit and have a cup of tea, so yeah, it's weird.

166

Needs Deprivation

It's important to note that these challenges in perspective taking do not imply a lack of empathy or an inability to understand others' emotions. Autistic individuals can still experience and express empathy, but they may have a different way of perceiving and interpreting social and emotional cues. It's also crucial to recognise that not all autistic individuals will have the same difficulties with perspective taking. Some autistic individuals may excel in certain aspects of perspective taking, particularly when it aligns with their specific interests or areas of expertise. Additionally, with support, practice and interventions, individuals with autism can develop and enhance their perspective-taking skills.

That said, perspective taking is two-sided and misunderstandings can also be two-sided (Heasman & Gillespie, 2017). Due to differences in neurocognitive processing, communication styles, processing information, expressing emotions and interpreting social cues, neurodiverse relationships experience the likelihood that misunderstandings will occur from each side. Any or all of these many differences and difficulties may be the cause of a needs deprivation for each in neurodiverse relationships and contributes, in part, to the unconventional features of these relationships.

Support Thoughts

It is important to note that in autistic-neurotypical relationships a significant needs deprivation will, more often than not, occur for both in these relationships and for NT people in particular. While mainly due to the function of different neurologies, initially it may be hard to ascertain. Owing to commonplace autistic behaviour kept hidden behind closed doors, along with the largely unknown but significant needs variances between the two types of people, the resulting unconventional relational patterns are unfamiliar to most people external to the relationship. Once understanding of these aspects occur, however, it will provide a framework to better support people in neurodiverse relationships.

Outcomes of living with a reality that is neither understood nor believed is discussed in the next chapter.

7

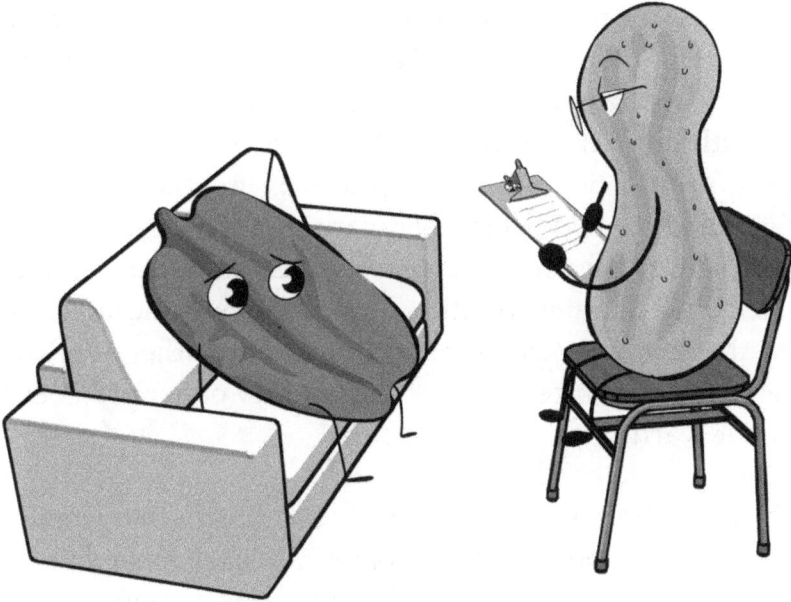

Heed Cassandra's Warning

Have We Gone Nuts?

**'Truth will always be truth, regardless of lack of
understanding, disbelief or ignorance.'**
W. Clement Stone

In Greek mythology, Cassandra was the daughter of
Priam, the last king of Troy, and his wife Hecuba. She was
considered the most beautiful of Priam's daughters but was not
a prophetess. According to Aeschylus's tragedy *Agamemnon*,
the god Apollo fell in love with Cassandra. Apollo provided
her with the gift of prophecy, but when Cassandra refused
Apollo's romantic advances, he placed a curse on her, ensuring
that nobody would believe her warnings. Apollo's cursed gift
to Cassandra became a source of endless pain and frustration
to her. She accurately predicted such events as the fall of Troy
and the death of Agamemnon but could neither alter these
events nor convince others of the validity of her predictions.
All her warnings went unheeded.

Today, the terms 'Cassandra', 'Cassandra Syndrome' or
'Cassandra Phenomenon' are sometimes used metaphorically
to describe those who make accurate predictions or warn
about potential dangers or problems but are disregarded or
dismissed by others. This can happen in various contexts,
such as in politics, economics, environmental issues or other
domains where warnings or concerns about future events may
be met with scepticism or apathy. Although many assume
that the Cassandra Phenomenon is restricted to women, it
can happen with any person.

In regard to neurodiverse relationships, the Cassandra
Phenomenon is sometimes said to arise when partners
or family members of people with ASC seek help but are

disbelieved (Rodman, 2003). Cassandra Phenomenon is also known as Cassandra Affective Disorder (CAD, Aston 2003), Cassandra Affective Deprivation Disorder (CADD, Aston 2003), Affective Deprivation Disorder (ADD; Simons 2009), or Post-Traumatic Relationship Syndrome (PTRS; Vandervoort & Rokach, 2004). Rodman (personal communication, 2010) has suggested that, when there is trauma in a relationship that has not ended, it should be referred to as Ongoing Traumatic Relationship Syndrome (OTRS) rather than PTRS. Yet, when it comes to neurodiverse relationships, the Cassandra terms have become very controversial.

Cassandra's Controversy

False impressions, much disagreement, and sometimes, outright hostility has developed over the use of the Cassandra terms. Many with ASC have mistakenly interpreted the Cassandra terms as putting all the 'blame' for all a relationship's dysfunction on the person with ASC. Some have also viewed the Cassandra terms as reflecting a prejudice against those with ASC (Simons & Thompson, 2009).

However, the struggles that NT people go through are not about being deliberately afflicted. It's more akin to being inadvertently deprived. Additionally, Simons and Thompson (2009) report that 'it is overly simplistic to say that one partner causes the deprivation of the other. Instead, the reality is that each partner may contribute to the dysfunction in different degrees' (p. 3).

It is the neurological differences between ASC and NT people that create a situation where people are emotionally out of sync with each other. When also considering the self-protective behaviours that autistic adults often engage in and their mindblindness (Baron-Cohen, 1997), the combination can contribute to a perception that the NT person in their lives is the source of relationship problems. Lacking an ability to distinguish the part they play in misunderstandings or difficulties may lead some people with ASC to inadvertently trigger symptoms of the Cassandra Phenomenon for their NT partner or family members. Rather than recognise their own contribution to difficulties, those with ASC may perceive they are being held liable for incidents of which they are entirely unaware, therefore innocent. Thus, the statements of their NT partners or family members are perceived as incorrect and therefore, not believed.

Jim (ASC) illustrated his unwitting need to avoid the conversations where he felt that Dianne (NT) 'gets fired up', where he 'gets disappointed in her behaviour' therefore, obviously he is innocent, and she should 'get over it'. However, in the process he completely missed that she was endeavouring to help him to 'try better' to interact with her to solve their problems:

> *She might see something that she is real fired up about, and I'm thinking 'Oh shit. Can't do anything about it, so forget about it' … So, as I said I just walk away. I don't bother … why hassle? I have got enough hassle in my life now without adding more. Yeah, I just get disappointed in her behaviour, but get over it. Got to. Well, that's all you can do, but the point is, okay it has happened get over it. The old saying, it's happened you can't do anything about it. Let's get over it and walk away. Build a bridge … She said, 'Well you should try' and I'm thinking, but try at what? You know, and this*

*is where the crux is. She said, 'Well you should be doing
something better.' Yeah, but ... what? And I'm thinking,
'Well okay fine.' I don't argue ... but for me when someone
says you should try more, yeah, well try at what? It's a big
question mark.*

Misunderstood in their relationships, many NT people
are also misunderstood for attempting to convey this
misunderstanding and explanations are contradicted as
misunderstandings and mistakes. When accompanied by
the dilemmas brought on by late diagnosis, self-diagnosis or
speculations of autism, the widespread complications of the
many unknowns of autism in adults may cause many NT
people to struggle to make sense of the distinct 'oddness' of
their relationships. Once coming to the realisation that autism
may be a consideration, they try to explain to others what
their life is like with an autistic partner or family member. Yet
their version of events is often questioned. The camouflaging
behaviour that many autistic people employ to conceal
differences, along with the unseen aspects inherent in autistic
behaviour which produces many of the unconventional
qualities to these relationships, may hide the facts of their
lives. As Tracy (NT) pointed out:

*James is a totally different person in public. I was cautious
enough not to tell any people whom I did not trust enough
to inform extensively.*

Despite the neurological differences and associated
problems in a neurodiverse relationship, the Cassandra
Phenomenon is not so much brought about by the emotional
deprivation that many NT people experience in their
relationship, but instead, it is created by the effect of not being

believed about their experience of emotional deprivation. Using the Cassandra terms are an attempt to describe this common NT experience.

Cassandra's Clues

Cassandra, therefore, is not about living with a mismatch of needs and expectations that arise from the interlocked misunderstandings and communication difficulties as Cassandra does not actually refer to the mismatch of needs and expectations themselves. Cassandra is also not about the experience of confusion that comes from having conventional expectations that a relationship would include mutual sharing of thoughts and feelings and then living with these expectations remaining unfulfilled. Cassandra is also not about conventional expectations of being able to experience relatively easy and effortless conversation about important topics and then living with these expectations continually remaining unfulfilled. Nor is Cassandra about the perplexing to understand and perplexing to describe clash of expectations and emotional needs. What Cassandra is actually about is the lack of belief in the truth of those experiences and the loneliness that results. It is the being dismissed. The being doubted. The feelings of isolation that follows. As such, Cassandra forms from being disbelieved and dismissed by the ASC people in a relationship, the others outside of a relationship and the resulting feelings of abandonment. An anonymous respondent (NT) described the pain of being disbelieved:

> Not being believed has been incredibly painful. If my partner has not personally experienced a similar event, it cannot be true.

Heed Cassandra's Warning

With little or no external support, the NT person is neither understood by their ASC partner/family members or by family, friends or professionals who could reasonably be thought to be empathetic. Thus, the total responsibility for the relationship often rests with them 'who report a feeling of "going mad", and who frequently become depressed' (Aston, 2002, p. 1). The lack of belief in their explanations, interpretations and feeling 'unheard' are what lays underneath the NT experiences of intense internal conflict, poor self-esteem, frustration, pent-up anger, rage, anxiety, depression and many other resulting health symptoms. In other words, the Cassandra Phenomenon.

Yet these feelings are often misunderstood as a criticism of autistic people. It is commonplace for people to fail to understand what is unknown to them. Accordingly, the fact that people tend to dismiss what appears to them as 'making a mountain out of a molehill' is understandable. However, in this instance, all is not as it first seems. Not looking at what lays beneath means a denial of the truth of the lives of those within neurodiverse relationships. Rae (NT) revealed her exasperation with inabilities to gain the understanding she needed:

> *My doctor told me to look up after Isaac had spent an hour with my psychologist, and she said, 'I think you'll find he has got Asperger's' and I said 'What!' Anyway, when I read it, I read that it said the hardest part for the spouse of an Aspie is to explain to their family and friends what it is like … Nobody gets it … and they wonder, they wonder why I am so angry all the time!*

Consequently, with limited community understanding of autism in adults, describing these facts to others are often batted away as misunderstandings and mistakes. Dismissed and disbelieved, often misunderstood in their relationship, most NT people have to endure ongoing doubts, questions, disregard and the inaccurate perceptions others hold. It is only natural for them to feel dissatisfaction, frustration and anger. This pent-up anger and frustration, however, may look to others as similar to blame and fault-finding. A side effect of the lack of recognition and support for being on the other side of adult autism. Yet it is the disbelieving and discounting of their experience that brings about their aggravation, not as an accusation against their loved ones, but as an accusation against the amount of distrust in their truth that they encounter. From their loved ones and from others.

The development of the Cassandra Phenomenon cannot be thought of as something that arises from solely being in a neurodiverse relationship, but it is from the isolation and loneliness of knowing a truth, experiencing that truth and the pain of not being believed (Simons & Thompson, 2009). Thus, the Cassandra Phenomenon highlights the need for recognition and support for NT people in neurodiverse relationships. Georgia (NT) stated that she noticed recognition gradually increasing:

> *I mean just being validated and knowing that its getting out there, people are starting to realise it's there, it happens, it's real and that the suffering, they call it like the Cassandra Phenomenon. Whether you call it the Cassandra Phenomenon or some sort of ongoing stress disorder you know like PTSD that kind of thing, we do suffer, we suffer as a consequence.*

Still, recognition is not always support or acceptance. With such limited research on adults with ASC, few studies have examined the features of Cassandra in neurodiverse relationships and the resulting impacts on individuals. Although a few studies have begun to turn the tide by mentioning the Cassandra Phenomenon or related terms (i.e. Arad, 2020; Bostock-Ling, 2012; 2017; Millar-Powell, 2020; Rench, 2014), the results have yet to filter through to clinicians and the wider population in general. As yet, the majority of information about the Cassandra Phenomenon is gained from anecdotal descriptions through personal accounts and therapists recommending strategies they have developed in their practices. Therefore, most literature currently used by clinicians to work with people in neurodiverse relationships is non-evidence based.

Through my research, I have endeavoured to reverse this situation. Using a 5-point Likert scale ranging from Always through to Never, participants in my study responded to two questions about being believed/not believed when describing relationship difficulties to others, such as family and friends or when seeking professional help regarding their relationship. These questions investigated a measure of belief/unbelief that participants experienced. The next section reveals some of participant responses.

A Need to Believe

In answer to survey statements and interview questions, many NT participants reported feeling anger and frustration at their inability to share the reality of their lives due to the lack of belief they regularly experienced. As previously discussed in Chapter 2, most participants reported that they found it too complicated to even begin to explain the unconventionality of their relationships, given that their lived experiences are mainly misunderstood and dismissed. When asked if she talked to family and friends about her relationship, Beth (NT) said, *'no because they don't understand'.*

Dealing with their situation alone, unable to reach out to others, the majority of NT participants reported feeling a sense of isolation, loneliness and powerlessness. The belief in their reports and the support that they anticipated from family and friends was not forthcoming. Dawn (NT) was surprised at the lack of acceptance of her husband's autism, even from people whom she thought would support her revelations:

My mother-in-law, who is ... a special needs teacher, she ... doesn't see it ... She was the one that went 'No he is not ... he is just going through a challenging period in his life.'

Likewise, Mandy (NT) found herself in a similar situation:

I did a lot of reading and research when we first met ... because I knew something wasn't right ... his father definitely has Asperger's and at least half of his brothers ... they just accept them as they are ... and his mother still won't have it that he's been diagnosed and he's got nephews now that are very young and the mothers are struggling because ... they just say, 'No there's nothing wrong with them, that's normal.' It's not normal. It's just accepted in that family as normal ... I spoke to him about it and brought it to his attention. Then he started to realise the things I was saying and the things I'd read were the things that he did and that's when we went and got diagnosed, so he understands it all well now, so we can talk about it.

Heed Cassandra's Warning

Aston (2003a) cites that many people in neurodiverse relationships feel 'misunderstood', while having their problems trivialised with many also being told that a partner's behaviour is 'simply being male' (p.11). Many NT participants discussed having these types of experiences:

WANDA   *Try to talk to friends or colleagues, its more 'Oh all men are like that' and I know that you've had that feedback before too, that you don't really feel that you're listened to or understood because they just … bring it all together as if oh that's just normal that's what all partners are like. Which isn't true at all. Or other people see your spouse as this, like you've seen his talent and he is able to communicate in a very professional manner to other people.*

TRACY   *A little bit of knowledge would, in my opinion, only lead to remarks such as, 'My husband is the same', or 'All men are like that'.*

QUINN   *In the beginning she was like, 'Well all the men are like that' or 'That's a man thing' … so, I started sending her information and she understands more now and she's more respectful of it now.*

WINNIE   *I did mention it to some people but they just come back with the usual, which I found out from the support groups, they said 'Oh no, he's just being a bloke and just being you know a blokey bloke.'*

Have We Gone Nuts?

MAGGIE   *I remember years ago I used to talk to people about my issues with Luke and the response would be 'Yeah, but my husband does that.' So, hence I have the problem, not him and so I pick and choose who I discuss it with.*

RENEE   *When I talked to friends about our situation you know the old phrase, 'Oh well that's just men' you know that sort of thing.*

Not only did they face a lack of belief and understanding, but the majority of NT participants also shared that they regularly had to deal with skepticism, cynicism and, at times ridicule when trying to explain the reality of their lives:

SOPHIE   *I usually do not [talk about my partner] because others have no concept of what I go through or deal with. The issues an NT partner of an AS man has, does not resemble anything from a normal NT–NT relationship for people to relate to. The few times I do reach out, usually it is when I forget people will not understand and their response quickly reminds me I shouldn't have reached out to them.*

RYAN   *I think a lot of her work colleagues, when I have met them, don't believe she is tricky to live with ... they sort of kind of think, 'Well what are you whining about?' ... If you are depressed, 'What's wrong with you?' ... Anything that reflects negatively upon me will be seen immediately as right by Rachelle's cousin because she's got no understanding of what Rachelle, what her personality is like, so yeah that's interesting!*

GEORGIA *I didn't get any support from my dad. My father just said, 'Oh well everybody has their problems'… and my husband loved that. He sort of stuck to my dad because my dad was very traditional. The man is the bread earner. The wife should just shut up and do what the man says … He just thought I was wrong and so I got no support from him, and I just shut my mouth and wouldn't talk to him … I wasn't believed that I was suffering and when you're rejected by your father, you're like, 'Well great! My husband behaves the way he does and I'm not getting the support I need from my dad.' That's tough in itself.*

QUINN *With my mum I've had conversations about him, I just don't ever say that I feel that he has a condition or whatever, you know, disorder and my mum can never understand … I haven't found that people are very understanding … haven't really been that helpful.*

MANDY *I said to him, 'Don't tell your mum that we've had it diagnosed', but he did, and she even comes to me sometimes and she'll say, 'He doesn't really have Asperger's. He's not on the spectrum. He doesn't have any sort of autism' and I'll say, 'Okay, alright' because there's no point. There's no point.*

181

Have We Gone Nuts?

NORA   *I don't feel people have the capacity or the space to understand what it's like being in a relationship with an Asperger's person ... people's general ability to process things is superficial.*

MAGGIE   *It's rather pointless ... They just don't get it. Other people don't get the subtlety of it and so you can't explain it so they're getting it all wrong and then they're telling you that you're the problem.*

LUCY   *And then the other problem we've got is they run off to people who they can trust to give them the answers they want. He goes to people like that and says, 'Oh Lucy thinks I'm Asperger. What do you think?' and they're like 'No.' Oh, it's so frustrating ... He said, 'Now look, I told [a friend] ... that you thought I was Asperger and he jumped on the net and said, "No!"' I said, 'You really think this is something that you can go to Dr Google on ... and decide that you weren't Asperger? I've been studying this for 3 years. Alice, my friend has been studying this longer because we really want things to be right. [Your friend] wouldn't know. You can't look at Dr Google and think you know Asperger. He doesn't know what goes on behind closed doors. He doesn't know you've already been ... that a psychologist in the field has unofficially diagnosed you'... He's got no comeback for that ... I rang his sister ... and I said, 'Look I'm walking away*

182

from him. I can't do this anymore' … He has spoken to her about it. She won't buy into the fact, yet she's done an Early Childhood University degree. Now she would have learnt about this … and she just says exactly what Pearce says, 'Oh, all relationships have their ups and downs.' But no, they have their ups and downs over something, not over nothing, and to me it makes me furious because what his own family are condoning is abuse, verbal and emotional abuse. He would never hit me, I would be shocked if he ever even raised his hand to me, that he's never done, it's all verbal and emotional … I said 'The bruises aren't on the outside, they're on the inside. That's where you leave them, Pearce.'

RENEE   *It's always so good to talk to somebody who absolutely knows. You don't have to explain. You try and explain this to, even family members … They just don't get it.*

Many also reported that they were written off as irrational:

HOLLY   *I've had one friend who gave me an absolute lambasting. She's, needless to say, no longer a friend, but she took me out after about a year and said to me. 'For goodness sake, pull yourself together. Jack's not the problem. You're the problem. You've just got to get over it', and every time she'd say, 'So what's he doing?' and I'd say, 'Such and such'. 'Oh, my husband does that', and so she just totally wrote off everything I said and then she said to me, 'Well it doesn't matter whether Jack's got something wrong with him or not, you've just got to get on with it', and she belongs to the 'pull yourself together' school of counselling and in the end I had no option. I had nowhere to go with her and I just had to say, 'Look, I'm really sorry that we're having a disagreement about this but it's pointless us continuing this conversation because you're not hearing how it is for me', and so I've chosen not to see her and that's a real sadness because I've lost friends over it.*

WANDA   *I think other women would challenge my sanity, like I haven't made any changes, yeah.*

RUTH   *It used to be that I was written off as 'emotional', 'crazy', or my thoughts and feelings about things just didn't make sense to him most of the time … I am selective about who I tell, though. I have had one friend who thought my husband's issue was me … My mother isn't always supportive, but she is likely on the spectrum too.*

RONDA   *Well, it's extremely hard because any of the dysfunction they see as coming from me. Just recently, like two weeks ago or three weeks ago I was Skyping with my second daughter who is married and has a child. She's in her 30s and I don't remember why I mentioned something about Asperger's, but she just really threw it back in my face and said, 'Oh it's not Asperger's. It's not that at all. In fact, he doesn't even have it. It's you that can't get along with anybody.' It's more than just being blamed, because everyone gets blamed for something unfairly in life. That is just part of life ... the difficult piece of that is other people seeing me as someone else and that is constantly being reflected not only from the Asperger partner 100% always, but from other people as well. And that constant reflection toward me for example from other people who know me when they project things that are not me. It's crazy making!*

While the majority of Cassandras are neurotypical, people on the spectrum can be Cassandras as well. Sandra (ASC) described the lack of belief in her and her son's diagnosis:

My dad and stepmum, when I've brought up things like ... my son diagnosed as being on the spectrum, they were just like, 'No he's not! ... It's ridiculous!' ... I've said to them a few times, 'You don't see all of it. You don't know everything that is going on' and that's when my stepmum will say, 'Well you don't tell us' ... a lot of it does have to do with because I feel like they're just going to dispute anything I say ... so I don't talk to them about much because I feel like they're going to be either judgemental or just be like, 'Well no. That's not what it is. That's not the case.' I guess I have heard that in the past before ... That's the way I cope with it, just not sharing information ... I do think I keep a lot back because I just don't want to hear an opposing side to it, so I just talk to my friends about it because they're not there to oppose anything.

This general lack of belief in their descriptions makes it virtually impossible for people in neurodiverse relationships to live in the truth of their situation, often leaving them with little option other than to hide their experiences. However, a major conundrum to hiding experiences for those with ASC, is that when autistic adults are able to accept themselves with recognition of a diagnosis, their health and happiness are likely to improve, and their relationships have a greater likelihood of success.

Although the data from my studies are based on neurodiverse relationships that consist of the NT/ASC combination, it is important to acknowledge that similar patterns have also been observed in the pairing of two autistic people. However, the study on marital satisfaction by Bolling (2015) found that the NT participants who were in relationship with a person on the spectrum were more distressed than their ASC/ASC counterparts. The Bolling (2015) study found that marital dissatisfaction over five scales: affective communication, problem-solving communication, time together, sexual dissatisfaction, and conflict over child rearing were all significantly higher for the NT/ASC participants than for the ASC/ASC participants.

My Cassandra Awakening

Walking past a church one day, I noticed a sign in their grounds. It read 'beware of half-truths, you might have the wrong half'. That saying has stayed with me. Many years later I discovered the principle behind that saying was to be more meaningful to me than I could have ever contemplated. Looking back to the time when my sister's act of vengeance changed my life with my ever-growing understanding, it gave me a bigger insight into how she had been able to fulfil her objective.

According to Redelmeier and Ng (2020), people tend to believe the first thing they hear because of a cognitive bias called the availability heuristic, which is a type of cognitive bias that helps us make fast, but sometimes incorrect, assessments and is 'defined as a tendency to judge the likelihood of a condition by the ease at which examples spring to mind' (p. 528). Rather than seeking out additional information to form a more complete and accurate understanding, the availability heuristic causes people to rely heavily on information that is easily available or noticeable to them. In other words, they may believe the wrong half of someone's half-truth if that half-truth was the first information they received.

Another reason that people may believe the first thing they hear is because they trust the person or source providing the information or have a lack of critical thinking skills. Seeking out multiple perspectives makes it easier to critically evaluate the information presented which has the potential to counter the wrong half of a half-truth. However, it does take effort, and many may choose not to make the effort, especially if it does not appear to be worth the effort.

Another feature to assuming an idea is correct is when it is repeated. Hassan and Barber (2021) state that 'repeated information is often perceived as more truthful than new information. This finding is known as the illusory truth effect, and it is typically thought to occur because repetition increases processing fluency. Because fluency and truth are frequently correlated in the real world, people learn to use processing fluency as a marker for truthfulness' (p. 1). This phenomenon was first identified in a study conducted at Villanova University and Temple University in 1977. In other words, when someone hears something repeated, even if a wrong half of a half-truth, it becomes more believable, the more times it is heard.

Therefore, information that is heard first and often is the information that is more readily accepted as true, even when additional information is presented that counters it. It dawned on me that these aspects of human reasoning have had a profound effect on my life. The difficult circumstances I found myself in with my sister all those years ago, with its dark residue of unbelief hanging over me, that still lingers to this day, has awakened in me the understanding that I have always been a Cassandra. Instead of trying to change minds, this Cassandra changed gears and moved towards investigation and understanding.

Support Thoughts

According to Dr Gurash, some professionals have begun to accept and understand the Cassandra Syndrome. We need many more. It is vital for professionals to be aware of the complex dynamics of neurodiverse relationships due to the differences in brain wiring. Many of the challenges found in these relationships are not typical. Those that do understand some of the differences, describe it as another experience that can contribute to relational trauma, also referred to as Complex PTSD. Complex PTSD is a form of trauma that doesn't occur from one singular big traumatic event but rather from a series of ongoing contextual trauma events through lack of intimacy, social connection, emotional deprivation and misattuned relationships (Gurash, 2023).

The experience of being in a relationship with someone on the spectrum who usually does not know how to acknowledge the feelings of others can be traumatising. Even when understanding that this behaviour is usually unintentional, it is also important to be aware that the impact on the mental and physical health of the NT person is the same, regardless. Therefore, neurodiverse relationships cannot be viewed in the same way as typical relationships. An understanding is required that atypical outcomes will result. The Cassandra Syndrome is one of many atypical outcomes.

According to Gurash (2023), behaviour that contributes to relational trauma may include:

- A lack of emotional connections and reciprocity
- Missing cues that you are feeling upset, misunderstood or ignored
- Trouble understanding your perspective of an experience
- Limited interpersonal skills
- Difficulty with communication
- Lack of empathy
- Challenges with reading your emotional experiences
- Difficulty regulating emotions

- Needing lots of time alone to decompress
- Lack of intimacy and emotional connection
- Symptoms of Cassandra Syndrome.

The misalignment in neurodiverse relationships can negatively impact the psychological and physiological symptoms of complex trauma and may include:

- Negative self-image
- Interpersonal challenges
- Anger and emotional regulation
- Anxiety and/or panic attacks
- OCD
- Hypervigilance; easily startled
- Social phobias
- Dissociation, flashbacks, and/or nightmares
- Physical illness and weakened immune system (Gurash, 2023).

Prior to developing interventions, it is important to understand what the problem is, what extent it must be addressed, and which outcomes could be improved. We look at some of the resulting negative impacts of low knowledge, misconceptions and myths about autistic adults and the subsequent effect on each in these relationships in the next chapter.

8

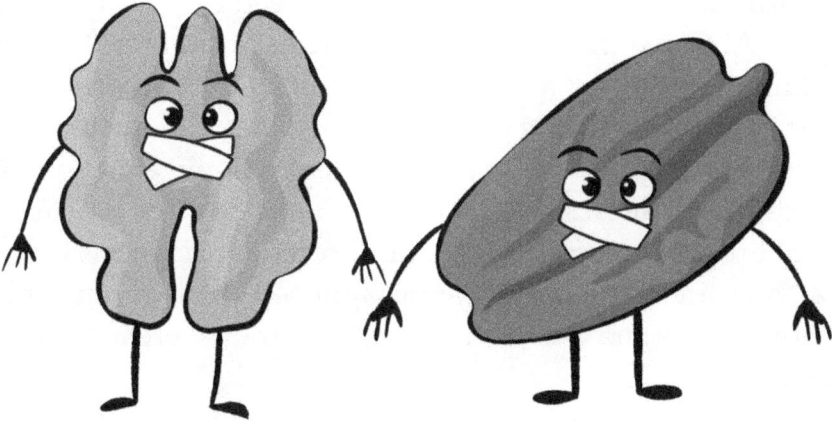

Conspiracies
of Silence

Have We Gone Nuts?

'Sometimes the strongest among us are the ones who smile through silent pain, cry behind closed doors, and fight battles that nobody knows about.'
Author unknown

Recent population-based studies estimate that at least 40% of primary-school age children who need to be diagnosed with ASC go unrecognised, resulting in many reaching adulthood without a diagnosis. When also considering the lost generation, that is those who are older adults, there are countless autistic adults who are living without a diagnosis, without understanding their differences and without support. While some autistic adults receive a diagnosis much later in life, some remain undiagnosed throughout their entire life. Some will never know that they were autistic.

A late diagnosis or coming to an understanding of autism and self-diagnosing later in life can be both validating and challenging. It can involve facing a unique set of experiences which are life-changing, such as directly questioning a sense of self, past narratives and future possibilities (Stagg & Belcher, 2019). It can also provide an explanation for lifelong experiences while at the same time presenting new challenges for self-education and managing autism or grappling with acceptance. However, concerns about disclosure, stigma and the need to camouflage contributes, in part, to the unconventional features of neurodiverse relationships as what is usually revealed to others does not make known the genuine set of circumstances behind closed doors.

Struggling with Stigma

Added to the challenge of adjusting to a new normal, there is the facing of a different kind of challenge: how others view ASC. Although a surge in research on ASC has led to some advances in understanding certain aspects, there continues to be a large focus on children, and as a result, few people have a concept of how autism manifests in adults. The resulting negative impact of low knowledge, misconceptions and myths about autistic adults often means that the decision on whether or not to disclose to others is not an easy one to make (Edwards et al., 2023). The dilemma of wanting increased understanding, acceptance, support or strengthened relationships has to be weighed up against potential exposure to being dismissed, judged or misunderstood. Shirley (NT) said:

> I think there's still a stigma around autism being a childhood disease. So, I can't stand it when I see things on the internet, on my news feed, social media around, you know like a video of an autistic couple 'Oh you know autistic people can be in relationships too'... I find it strangely offensive that it's even a conversation. I would like to see it become less stigmatised ... I'd like to see heaps more stuff in the media about autistic adults and the contributions they make to our society, which is just outstanding and ... just reduce that stigma around how autistic people can't be in romantic relationships. I know it's still out there. In our circles we don't hear it much, but it is out there, so that would be good if it became a little bit more ... accepted, or more like widespread, like more in the media.

Since most masked autistic adults have struggled for decades before discovering who they truly are, they usually choose not to divulge this newfound knowledge to others.

Have We Gone Nuts?

Research has confirmed that the majority of families with autistic children, as well as the majority of autistic adults experience reservations about disclosure (Han et al., 2023; Kinnear et al., 2016). They mostly feel that it will be a negative experience or create problems. One of the main reasons is the fear of stigma. According to Bos et al. (2013) stigma involves a recognition of difference and devaluation and includes a fundamental dimension of the degree to which these aspects can be concealed.

A study by Kinnear et al. (2016) found that almost all of the families with autistic children felt that individuals with autism are stigmatised. However, the fear of being stigmatised is usually felt more acutely by adults. A study by Edwards et al. (2023) concluded that 'autistic adults feel the impact of society's lack of understanding of autism on a daily basis whether they disclose or not, with widespread stigma and experiences of discrimination across contexts such as employment, health care and relationships, with these experiences reducing their quality of life' (p. 10). There is also evidence that stigma is linked to poorer mental health in autistic adults. Despite this, choosing to hide a stigmatised condition and attempting to 'pass' as 'normal', has the potential to create even more stress. It places people in the position of continually living with the fear of being discovered as well as ongoing anxieties regarding who they should tell. Both these responses are significant sources of psychological distress (Bos et al., 2013).

My study concluded that although stigma is often entrenched in misconceptions, stereotypes and the lack of understanding about autism in adulthood, the deficit narrative that is so prevalent about autism, means that 'pretending to be normal' or camouflaging autism was the preferable option that most participants chose. Rather than disclosing to others, they tended to adopt the stance of keeping a socially accepted façade. This façade was a construct that both ASC and NT participants endeavoured to uphold, and in public both ASC and NT participants tried to appear like a 'normal' family and/or couple. Samuel (ASC) described the sense of normalcy that his pretending everything was 'normal' gave to him:

I can't provide her with what she needs in the relationship because of my Asperger's ... We have the kids' girlfriends' parents over at night and we just act like any other normal couple. Dinner is made. We sit down and drink wine and chat. I get to have a family ... So, we're getting things from it. It's just not your standard relationship that's all. So yeah, we just get on with it, we've got our friends, no-one really says anything, they just come and visit, and we act like a couple and it's all good, yeah.

On the other hand, a study by Sasson and Morrison (2019) found that 'diagnostic disclosure helps rather than harms social evaluation of adults with ASD, particularly when peers have knowledge about the characteristics of autism' (p. 55). Their study found that when people are told of a diagnosis of autism, negative perceptions of the behaviours associated with autism are lessened. Therefore, contrary to popular belief, a diagnostic label can provide people with an explanation for what they perceive to be atypical social behaviour and this explanation often influences a more positive attitude towards the person, especially when given the opportunity to understand autism.

Hiding in Plain Sight

Camouflaging, also known as 'masking', refers to the practice of hiding or suppressing autistic traits and behaviours in social situations. It can be used consciously or unconsciously by mimicking or imitating social behaviours, communication styles and other aspects of NT behaviour in order to fit in and appear more non-autistic. While this behaviour is often employed as a coping mechanism to navigate social situations, make friends and maintain relationships, it is also used to overcome the fear of stigma.

However, camouflaging autism can cause many other lasting problems for autistic adults. It can be emotionally and mentally exhausting, leading to burnout, anxiety and a sense of identity loss. It can delay a diagnosis which can hinder access to appropriate support and accommodations. It can mean that autistic adults may feel the need to hide their true selves to maintain employment or sustain a relationship, which can be emotionally taxing. It can cause challenges in advocating for their needs and raising awareness about autism because they appear to be 'high-functioning' and may not fit the stereotype of autism. It may mean having to decide when it is necessary to mask traits and when to be authentic. This decision-making process can be exhausting.

While camouflaging primarily affects autistic adults, it can also have a significant impact on their NT partners and family members. Many NT participants described how their partners and family members' camouflaging behaviour caused a rift between their private and public lives:

RAE   *People say, 'But what do you argue about?'*
Because in public Isaac seems, such you know
'Mr Congeniality'... Everybody just thinks
he is so lovely. Everybody just loves Isaac ...
He's the perfect gentleman and he's not nasty
and of course when other people see him, he's
jovial ... when they see him socially, they say
'everybody loves Isaac'... 'What do you fight
about?' and I thought, 'I can't even begin to
tell you. I can't even put it into words,' because
that sort of interaction doesn't happen when
you are out socially.

HALEY   *In public ... it was what was socially acceptable,*
so he would always come and put his arm
around me, and I used to think, 'Well you
can't any other time, but you come and make
out that we are really close' ... When we were
in public, he would make a big effort like it
was important because 'this is my wife sort
of thing'. It was all about ... the image, it's all
about what is perceived to be the right thing.

TRACY   *At first, I did not dare to tell anyone because*
I honestly thought I must be doing something
wrong and that with patience, love and time,
things would work out. Only when they did
not, did I confide in a friend ... because James
is a totally different person in public.

WINNIE   *You can't talk, I don't talk to my family, and*
I don't talk to my friends about it ... they just
couldn't see what I could see ... so the façade

Have We Gone Nuts?

and the persona that he puts on in public ...
when we come home that just all falls away.

Paradoxically, while camouflaging is an attempt to fit in socially, it can lead to social isolation. The effort to mask autistic traits may make it difficult for individuals to form genuine connections with others. While this is true for all relationships, when a lack of disclosure together with unresponsiveness are added, the combination can be detrimental to the development of intimacy in close relationships.

Confirmed by research, the links between camouflaging, autistic identity and disclosure about being autistic has a huge impact on the mental health of autistic people (Cage & Troxell-Whitman, 2020). Additionally, long-term camouflaging can make it difficult for adults to understand and accept their true selves because they have spent so much time pretending to be someone they are not. This can negatively impact their relationships with their partners and family members. Laurenceau et al. (1998) found that self-disclosure, other disclosure and other responsiveness, at an interaction-by-interaction level were the most significant components to the formation of closeness and intimacy between people, while Webster et al. (2009) add that expressing closeness on an intimate level encourages an equivalent response in others. People generally reciprocate others' level of disclosure, whether the source is a romantic partner or a stranger. In support of this concept, Derlega (2013) and Mashek and Aron (2004) report that, without disclosure and responsiveness, it can become difficult to love a person when that person is difficult to get to know in a more meaningful and connected way.

In addition, a study by Cage and Troxell-Whitman (2020) found that while the decision to disclose involves evaluating who, what, when and how much to disclose, people who were able to be more openly autistic, camouflaged their autism less than those who were not openly autistic. Their study also found that in situations where nondisclosure was the safest option, especially from fear of stigma, people became trapped in an internal conflict between the need to declare their autistic identity and the fear of discrimination, which led to becoming resigned to use camouflaging. Rachelle (ASC) agreed with this sentiment as she expressed her irritation at feeling required to camouflage her autism:

> *I feel like I'm faking it every day and I can't be the person I want to be … I just have to conform to what society wants me to be and I can't talk to people the way I want to talk to people. I have to put in all these nice words and use inflection in my voice and try and act normal … People think I'm rude … and I'm just surrounded by people who aren't on the spectrum, at work and with my husband … It's like being from another planet, speaking another language and yeah, it's difficult. It's like I wake up every day and when I leave the house I have to put on a mask and pretend … when we see other people communicating and smiling at each other and chatting away … the small talk, it's all fake like it's all just nothing, meaningless, we don't find any meaning in it … it looks meaningless.*

Anonymous survey respondents (ASC) agreed with this sentiment:

> *I have learnt to pretend to be neurotypical, but it mostly works outside of our relationship.*

Have We Gone Nuts?

I have had so much therapy and social skills training, that I now go through the motions to get on with people, and wear an invisible mask each day, and do things that aren't authentic, to keep everyone else happy and get ahead in life. Do I believe what I am doing? No! I don't believe it. It is important to other people, so I am faking it. It is important to other people to take turns, so I do it. I don't believe it as something important to me, rather it is something important to other people that I fake because I want something out of that other person (information, speed in processing my request, etc).

The study by Cage and Troxell-Whitman (2020) highlight 'the difficult process for autistic people in terms of weighing up the costs and benefits of disclosing or camouflaging in different contexts' (p. 337). Therefore, it is important to provide ways in which autistic people can be supported to be able to 'take the mask off' so that our communities can become discrimination-free. In order for this to happen there needs to be a change in how society views autistic adults so that they can have the freedom to choose to disclose their autistic identity, because doing so can help to reduce the need for camouflaging (Cage & Troxell-Whitman, 2020). This change will not only support autistic adults, but also their partners and family members as well.

Consequently, regardless of the upsurge of autism research, matters of stigma and disclosure surrounding autism is still a significant challenge for people with ASC, for their partners and for their families. Clearly, it is vital to change how society thinks and acts towards autistic people (Han et al., 2023). Until then, the risks involved in disclosure may mean the majority of autistic adults may want to continue to mask their autism, even when privately aware of a different reality. Understanding these issues are essential for developing targeted supports and interventions, both for those with autism and their partners and family members.

Support Thoughts

Whether clinician, counsellor, autistic person or a family member or friend of an autistic person, making it a priority to gain knowledge about adult autism is necessary to become a more autism friendly and autism understanding community. When society is able to be more supportive and less judgemental of autistic adults and their partners and families, it will allow them to come out from behind closed doors, break free from the conspiracies of silence and openly declare being autistic or in a neurodiverse relationship. This will go some way towards supporting and accommodating the needs of autistic adults and their partners and family members and contribute to creating more inclusive and supportive environments for autistic people and their significant others.

Addressing the dilemma of camouflaging adult autism involves recognising the challenges it poses and providing support, acceptance, and accommodations to autistic individuals. It's crucial for society to foster an environment where neurodiversity is celebrated, and individuals are encouraged to be their authentic selves without fear of judgement or rejection. Additionally, healthcare professionals and educators should be trained to recognise the signs of camouflaging and provide appropriate guidance and resources for autistic adults so that they can feel free to reveal their true selves without the fear of stigma. The effect of these challenges on the delivery of support and/or services for those in neurodiverse relationships is discussed in the next chapter.

9

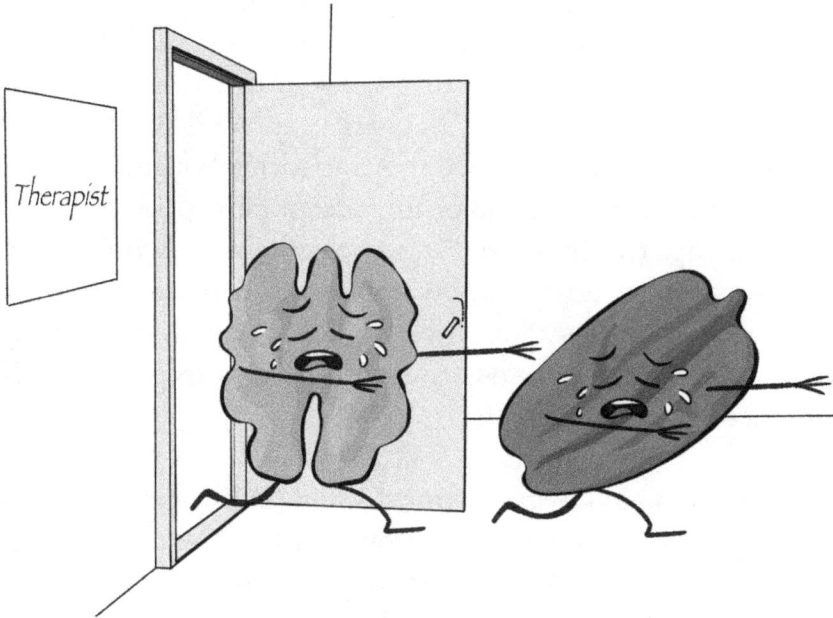

Clinical
Complications

Have We Gone Nuts?

**'Don't base your decisions on the advice of those
who won't have to deal with the results.'**

Anonymous

Given that very little research has been conducted in
relation to adults on the autism spectrum and even less has
been conducted in relation to their close relationships, there
is a gap in evidence regarding these adults in general and
neurodiverse relationships in particular. While this gap has
allowed numerous misconceptions to form about adults with
ASC, it has also had a major impact on perceptions of their
relationships (Rodman, 2003). As a result, many who provide
support and/or services know very little about autistic adults
and know even less about their relationships. Consequently,
the majority of clinicians are not trained or experienced in
diagnosing ASC in adults.

According to Lai and Baron-Cohen (2015), it is often only
those with more severe symptoms, such as extreme social
aloneness, no eye contact, and frequent motor mannerisms,
or those with concurrent developmental difficulties, such
as cognitive or language delay, that tend to receive an early
diagnosis. For adults who do not present as stereotypically
autistic, such as those who would have previously been
identified with AS, those with more subtle difficulties, or those
who are unaware of their condition, may go unrecognised
until later life, if at all (Lipinski et al., 2019; Lipinski et al.,
2021; Smith & Jones, 2020; Strunz, 2018). Yet, Mendes (2015)
estimates that up to 50% of adults with ASC are undiagnosed
or misdiagnosed, but it is quite likely that the percentage is
much higher. Anonymous survey responses illustrate some
of the challenges of obtaining a diagnosis:

Jake was 13 when he was diagnosed with high functioning ASD. If we had a diagnosis a lot earlier, when we knew he was different at 4 years of age, it would have been easier to understand his behaviour and assist him. We have seen many Speech Pathologists, Psychiatrists, Therapists and Psychologists during his life and feel that they let us down by not providing an accurate diagnosis.

It is almost impossible in regional Australia to get a diagnosis, and treatment by medication is a hit and miss response. Often drugs are prescribed which lead to addiction and psychotic episodes. Getting to see someone like Attwood in Brisbane is a 2-year wait. My son is now 32 and my cry is for help. I have a PhD in History and have taught at many universities … but have been unable to contribute for 20 years because of the lack of understanding of my son's problems.

After years of frustration a therapist finally diagnosed my spouse with Asperger's and that has made a very big difference in what I expect in our relationship. The anxiety level has decreased for both of us. I have stopped expecting a NT relationship and look for the good qualities that are in our relationship.

Too Little Too Late

A report by Anon (2020) states that autistic adults 'experience significant difficulties in forming and maintaining long-term relationships with friends, family, co-workers and intimate partners, but without the support the younger generation is currently receiving' (p. 1). Lacking the benefit of early intervention, growing up unaware of their condition, and experiencing society's misunderstanding, the adults of today, together with their partners and family members, are often required to face obstacles they have little knowledge of how to manage. Fiona (NT) lamented the lack of services for adults:

I wish that there was a service for adult Asperger's people, whereas there are a lot of services and support for children but there are none for adults. And child Asperger's people become adult Asperger's people. It doesn't go away ... With the support training that child Asperger's people have now, they are better equipped, I would theorise, to cope with an NT world than the adult Asperger's ... people because they never had that childhood support or understanding and tuition ... People like William has had to fumble through life learning by themselves without any basis for understanding the world that they are living in and I reckon that their parents didn't know anything about it anyway so they couldn't give the support.

Cora (ASC) agreed with this sentiment, wishing that she had known much earlier:

I wish ... that someone gave me information ... early on ... It would have helped me a lot to know ... sooner. I wouldn't have blamed myself ... He led me to believe I was always at fault and shattered my self-esteem.

A Counselling Calamity

Since most clinicians and healthcare professionals went through their education at a time when autism was mainly unknown, they have little to no experience in recognising autism in adults and often do not know how to work with neurodiverse couples. Therefore, psychologists and counsellors only know how to use methods that do not work in the context of these relationships (Anon, 2020; Lipinski et al., 2021). Holly (NT) spoke about how unsuitable regular counselling was for her husband:

And Jack was going for a lot of counselling on his own, supposedly to get back with me, but in actual fact he was just resting on his laurels, and I don't think ... the neurotypical counselling was being received or integrated into his life because he can't.

Not able to achieve the understanding or specialised help that they require, adults in neurodiverse relationships are often obligated to bear the responsibility of this lack of awareness themselves. Left to carry an undue burden of 'being invisible' and 'unheard' they often have little chance of finding appropriate support to ease the burden. Katy (NT) agreed with this sentiment:

It's rare that you find a counsellor that really understands.

Aston (2003a) reports that at least 75% of neurodiverse couples seek counselling, but the majority are dissatisfied with the service and the resultant effects on their relationships. Mitran (2022) concurs, giving details that the use of cognitive behavioural therapy (CBT), a frequent therapy used for a person with high levels of anxiety and hypervigilance, as is common in the AS community, can sometimes result in exacerbated anxiety. Accordingly, when trying to seek counselling to help with relationship difficulties, the majority in neurodiverse relationships are subjected to counter-therapeutic practices. Both ASC and NT participants reported dissatisfaction with the professional services that was available to them. William (ASC) described the long journey he and Fiona (NT) had been on to try and find appropriate assistance, but without much success:

Yeah well, we went to [a psychologist] ... That didn't work. I was so distressed ... I got told that I'm just pretending ... I firmly believe that the way I act, and think is to do with early experiences to a great extent. The theory of complex PTSD ... But that doesn't seem to be recognised, or taken a lot of notice of, by a lot of psychologists ... I saw a psychologist once a long time ago. He wasn't much use ... Anyway, gave him up. We went to a marriage counsellor psychologist. She was a homely sort of person; I thought this might just suit us. A bit older and she didn't have much to offer either ... Her advice ended up being that 'One doesn't say the things which would upset the other.' Which on the surface sounds okay, but when you've got psychological triggers involved, it's much more complex ... Anyway, the thing is to find someone who can mediate. Not only that, but can understand that to some extent and give that sort of advice ... The psychologist we've been to now, he says, 'Oh yeah, Asperger's is most likely', but he's more or less ignoring that we're dealing with two people. We're going to do behaviour modification, cognitive, CBT... It should probably be both, but that sort of therapy is usually only reserved for the Asperger person because we need changing. Well, you can't change.

Haley (NT) reported a lack of success, even with a specialist who was supposed to have appropriate knowledge:

The last lady we went to, I didn't think she was as good as she could have been to help him understand and work through things, and she was supposed to ... specialise in Asperger's. But whether it wasn't a good thing he wasn't diagnosed ... she would never sort of discuss anything like that with me. I would say to her, 'Well does he show the traits of someone with it?' And she goes 'Oh, I can't really talk', and she would want to talk about me. And I thought, 'Well I am here to try and save my marriage.'

Quinn (NT) described her attempts to seek out help, but also with little success:

I have twice. The very first time the lady made us face each other and tell us the things that bother us. She wasn't an Asperger's; she wasn't even a psychologist. She was a counsellor, so I don't think she would have been able to help us anyway, but he didn't like the way, it was kind of uncomfortable the way that she approached the situation, so we didn't go back and then I tried it one more time with a gentleman and ... that didn't go anywhere else either ... We haven't found anybody local that can help us. There's no-one other than that clinic that we thought could help and then the clinic, it sounds like, all they do is give you the diagnosis and then maybe a list of resources and you're on your own again. So, it wasn't what we expected.

Research has confirmed that many autistic adults experience comorbid psychological diagnoses such as anxiety or depression, yet 'psychotherapists' lack of knowledge and expertise seem to be a major barrier for adults with autism to receiving helpful psychotherapeutic support' (Lipinski et al., 2021, p. 1509). An anonymous survey response illustrates the ongoing struggle that a lack of helpful psychotherapeutic support produces in people's lives:

> [There are] real difficulties obtaining marriage counselling by counsellors aware of Asperger's and when counsellors are identified, very hard to be able to get appointments, which when coupled with a reluctance on the part of my Asperger's partner to go to counselling in the first place, means very little real prospect of us ever dealing with the issues in our relationship in a constructive way.

Lucy (NT) reported that, rather than receive effective help, the psychologist visits had made things worse:

> I ended up with a psychologist … so he ended up spending a year with her and she was treating him for anger management. The common thread here anybody who just goes, if they're Asperger, and they go to a normal psych it just makes it worse. I've since written to her just recently, I just said 'Look if anybody presents like this again, you told him in front of me that a habit could be broken in three months.' He was with her for 12. 'And you cut him loose because you were making no impression on him, and it didn't even twig at all that there was something else going on.' … She did respond to me and said, 'Thank you', for bringing it to her attention, because I said, 'Look I'm writing to you in the hope that if somebody presents like him to you again, that you'd take a deeper look.' It's like a GP doing brain surgery. It's not going to happen!

Dealing with Doubts

The ramifications of lack of recognition of adult autism in the community are wide-ranging. At the same time as facing the challenge of coming to terms with what a diagnosis or self-diagnosis means for their lives, many in these relationships also have to contend with being doubted by the very people who ought to provide support and/or services. When their specific difficulties are denied by others, it can hinder their ability to make consistent headway with their emerging understanding. It can also hinder their ability to work through their difficulties with others. Cora (ASC) described the disbelief many professionals exhibit:

Yes. I saw a CBT specialist in London, when we were living there, but I stopped seeing her because she had no understanding of ASD and insisted, I didn't have it. Her knowledge was very poor. She thought only men and boys got it and I should have 'ticks' and communicate poorly, and such.

Terry (ASC) described a similar experience:

We've been through a number of psychologists ... I went to one psychiatrist who just didn't believe it, and I referred to some of the other people that I'd seen which included Tony Attwood and just about any adult with a diagnosis of Asperger's pretty well knows who Tony Attwood is, I think because of the books and the papers that he's been involved with and the support that he's given to other psychologists in this country and around the world and he'd never heard of him so he sort of wasn't sure about this diagnosis. Yeah, I think I only saw him two or three times and decided no that wasn't going to work for me because I think he thought that I was not on the spectrum because ... I tried to be open and honest and establishing communication right from the word go ... I knew that if I just sat there and listened to him I wasn't going to benefit out of it.

An anonymous respondent (NT) also described a similar experience:

Communication problems were at the heart of all our marital difficulties. Over 33 years of marriage we never resolved a single issue. When told this fact, counsellors told me that I was lying, that it wasn't possible. The only way we resolved any issue was if it was so minor that neither of us really cared about the result, or by my – the NT – giving in, even if it did matter. Ultimately this was damaging to my self-esteem.

Dawn (NT) revealed:

I found this woman who said that she knew about autism, and I went to her and just vented 45 minutes and at the end of it she said, 'I think he has a mood disorder.' I didn't feel the need to go back again.

Most NT participants discussed the difficulties involved in navigating the doubts they received due to a lack of knowledgeable professionals:

MANDY   *I sent him to the doctor to talk to them about the fact that that's what I thought, and I had a doctor tell him that Asperger's was a children's disorder. Yeah, really helpful!*

Clinical Complications

SHIRLEY   *I would tend not to talk to a professional about our relationship problems unless they have extensive experience in autism. It's just the ignorance, like if I tried to explain to a psychologist who has had no contact with autistic people or no learning about autism and if they got a glimpse into how Jill and I, like they wouldn't understand. I don't think they would be in a position to sort of offer some really helpful advice, so we pay a lot of money to see someone who is quite a specialist in autism, yeah.*

RENEE   *I went to our GP ... when I brought this stuff up, he really kind of dismissed it you know, he basically said to me ... 'What difference does it make?' ... It makes a huge difference, but I suppose from his point of view ... there probably wasn't a lot of information available and here was somebody coming to him saying, 'Well I think my husband has this', and again that was like, 'Well no!' ... That kind of stuff then is reinforced, this whole thing about not knowing what I'm talking about. Not knowing anything and that was reinforced by Patrick not really knowing who I am and all of that sort of stuff so ... your own observations and things don't actually matter because you're just a mother who doesn't really know anything. But anyway, don't go down that track!*

BETH   *I would definitely not go to a GP and talk to them about this.*

213

Have We Gone Nuts?

DIANA   *We'd been shipped from one specialist to another and at one stage my husband had been violent. His brother took us up to the hospital and the doctor there, kind of well, you know about just having to control your emotion and anger and whatever else. And I asked this doctor if he could write down what he'd said because my husband has trouble remembering things and he said, 'Oh well, you look like a decent fellow. You'll remember this conversation when you know.' And that was the doctor up at the hospital who didn't take anything seriously whatsoever. And then we had another psychologist that was rather similar, 'It just sounds like a communication problem. I don't know why you're here to see me.' And that was that ... but yeah in the past we've had paramount problems I suppose with health professionals.*

RUTH   *We went to regular marriage counselling with a pastor... but didn't understand the root of the issues or seem to get that my husband lacked common sense, empathy, and the ability to see my perspective on anything. He did seem to get that my husband was immature and focused on himself. He made comments like, 'I'm pretty sure he can handle that', in reference to some parenting things and dressing the kids appropriately for the weather, etc., and I just shook my head. 'No.'*

214

Clinical Complications

Maxine Aston reports that untrained therapists can also be deceived by someone who gives the appearance of being very articulate, is usually very intelligent, has a good job and does not understand why his/her NT partner is never happy (Aston, 2003b). According to Aston (2003b), a counsellor can then unwittingly reinforce ASC behaviour and consequently reinforce the Cassandra Phenomenon. Many NT participants recounted this type of experience:

MAGGIE   *I think this is scary. We went to couples counselling with a psychologist that was supposed to know about AS and ... you hope professionals will get it ... because being a counsellor I realise how important it is to actually be aware of AS when people come in for counselling. I always felt that the psychologist actually sided with Luke so if you get a professional that actually understands AS then they side with the AS because the AS has the problem and I have to work around. This is how I felt. I have to do all the work to work around his AS and I was talking to her about the ... day in day out nothing ever being put away, nothing ever being resolved, nothing ever being fixed, nothing ever being done. Day in, day out for 30 years just about. Sends your head round the bend, and she talked to Luke, 'Oh well, Luke you could do blah, blah, blah. You could do that couldn't you?' And he goes, 'Oh yeah', and so that was the end of that. He could do that, but he never did do that ... but what she said to me, which made me react, she turned around and she said, 'Oh well maybe we need to look at some changes that you will have to make Maggie', and the hair stood up on the back of my neck and I was really angry and I leant forward and I just said to her, 'You don't live with him.' I was really angry and to me she didn't get how it affected me. The professionals need to understand how it affects both parties, not just one.*

WANDA   *Always not believed. If we go to see the psychologist that he sees who specialises with people on the spectrum, she does understand it, but it's also if we go see her together which we've been a few times, more recently, I always feel that he has the last word or if I say something that might be challenging, he'll give his explanation and you sort of have to go with that.*

Additionally, an often-overlooked characteristic of adults with ASC is the lengths that they will often go through to avoid a change that they do not want to make, both in themselves and in their circumstances. While this desire for sameness is central to the condition, sometimes it can have a negative impact on accessing professional help. It is important to note that this desire for sameness is often driven by fear. After a lifetime of doing things a certain way which feels comfortable and correct, it can be fearful to change, which triggers resistance. Laura (NT) mentioned her partner's resistance put a stop to the potential to achieve support for them both:

Clinical Complications

He wouldn't participate. Contemptuous of psychiatry, and what is there to work on, anyway!

The fear factor is important to keep in mind when dealing with resistance to change. Recognising that fear is a possible driver, can make it more understandable and make dealing with resistance a lot easier. Although William (ASC) spoke about his resistance, he made a profound point:

Nah, I deal with it myself. Don't need it. I tried it a couple of times and it winds up being an intellectual challenge between me and the counsellor, and I always win. In my opinion. No when we've done the counselling bit ... all the talking and counselling in the world, which is what Fiona is inclined to go along with, at the end of the day it is my decision as to how I deal with things, what I listen to, and what I do and if there is any changes to be made I need to do it. And I think it is whether I want to change.

Anonymous survey responses demonstrated that a knowledgeable therapist could make a difference:

Been in therapy for a few months now and discovered my ASD and have the problem of communication that builds up in me and need to let it out as soon as possible to not have a regrettable outcome of emotional hurt to my wife. Since the discovery I have of ASD I feel I woke up from a coma, and now on a journey of healing of 65 years of not knowing this about myself.

My diagnosis of Asperger's has only come within the last two months. So, I am still learning how to navigate through this world armed with this new knowledge and the help of my psychologist.

Support Thoughts

Smith et al. (2020) suggest neurodiverse relationships be regarded as 'intercultural relationships' (p.3318) due to the unique communication challenges that manifest. Through this lens, intervention strategies should focus on supporting couples to understand each other's cultures and, together, develop solutions to resolve differences in communication and social strategies (Tili & Barker, 2015). Aston (2003a) suggests several strategies for working with people in neurodiverse relationships impacted by ASC, including assessing the autistic partner's availability for counselling, clearly establishing that counselling will not transform inherent characteristics of autism and an acceptance that the majority of changes will need to be implemented by the NT partner through aligning the language of the couple. This includes direct, clear and concise verbal communication that lacks elements such as sarcasm, innuendo and double meaning. Just as importantly, counsellors must encourage both parties to develop a mindset that is willing to learn about each other's neurological differences. Awareness that neurological differences are often the basis for disagreements may defuse resulting conflict.

In the next chapter we continue the discussion on the counter-therapeutic practices that often result from the lack of understanding of the particular nuances that ASC brings to a relationship.

10

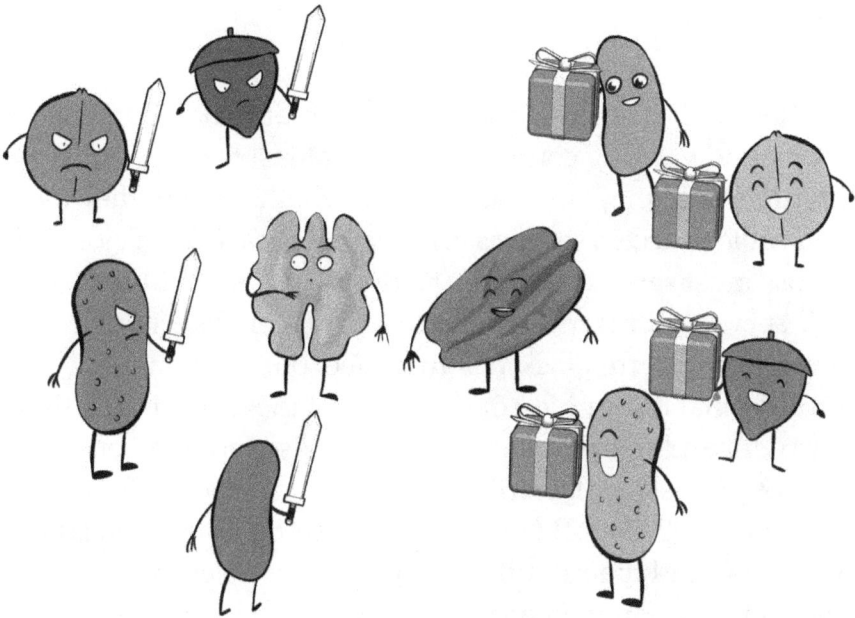

A Double-Edged
Sword

Have We Gone Nuts?

**'He that gives good advice, builds with one hand;
he that gives good counsel and example, builds
with both; but he that gives good admonition
and bad example, builds with one hand and pulls
down with the other.'**
Francis Bacon

Research has shown that although autistic people have many and varying complex needs that last throughout their lifetime, once they reach adulthood, whether or not they have been able to access services, they usually reach a 'service cliff' across most service systems (Koffer Miller et al., 2018). While this service cliff is mostly due to a persistent lack of research on adults and this lack has impeded both community and professional recognition of the needs of these adults and their partners and family members, it has also led to a continual lack of professional training. In a study conducted by Koffer Miller et al. (2018), all participating staff together with adults with ASC and their families, all testified wholeheartedly that the lack of appropriate training of professionals had led to devastating consequences for them and that it ought to be a top priority to reverse the situation. My studies confirmed a similar participant sentiment.

Koffer Miller's study also identified another complication regarding professional training. Since there are immense gaps in knowledge about autism in adulthood, a whole constellation of training is required across multiple different fields for professionals to fully grasp the reality of the situation. As it stands there is a lack of resources, a lack of program development and a lack of appropriate interventions to properly support autistic people, their partners and their family members across the continuum of their various needs (Koffer Miller et al., 2018).

A way that professionals can begin to appreciate the unconventional features of neurodiverse relationships is to revise their perspectives by concluding that it is essential to seek out quality training. Neurodiverse relationships are distinctive. They cannot be compared to conventional relationships. Smith et al. (2020) suggest that neurodiverse relationships be considered as 'intercultural relationships' (p. 3318) due to the unique challenges they experience. This interpretation may assist professionals to gain a better understanding of how to support the needs of both ASC and NT people when in a relationship together (Smith et al., 2020). Although framing neurodiverse relationships as intercultural serves as a way to work on the issues that result from a non-apparent disability without pathologising people, still, an extensive understanding of autism in adulthood is paramount in order to fully address the gaps in knowledge about their particular needs and support all concerned in these relationships.

Just as importantly, this intercultural interpretation can provide a tangible framework for people in neurodiverse relationships. Not only does this interpretation illustrate how distinctive neurodiverse relationships can be, but it can also enable people in these relationships to better understand the distinctiveness of their relationship structure. It may also help them to implement strategies to maintain or change their relationship (Smith et al., 2020). However, Wally (ASC) said:

Have We Gone Nuts?

I have a lot of friends who are in intercultural marriages where they've learned how to deal with their really significant cultural differences. I have one couple who we're good friends with, she's Japanese, he's Iranian ... and they still manage to communicate.

Slim Pickings

In light of the lack of community understanding and insufficient support avenues, participants in my studies were asked to detail the limitations that they had found with service providers for neurodiverse relationships. The majority of both ASC and NT participants indicated that the few services that did have knowledge of their particular difficulties were either, challenging to find and often inadequate when located, were too expensive for them, or were not within a distance close enough to access on a regular basis. Terry (ASC) described that while good progress had occurred at the beginning of some of his therapy sessions, he found it to be short-lived:

She was very good at getting me to open up and present certain ideas and perhaps how to stop doing something and replace it with something else but again we got to a particular stage where after probably 6 to 8 months I was seeing her that I wasn't getting any further progress with her.

Very few NT participants reported having a good experience when consulting with medical practitioners, therapy providers or when in counselling situations. As previously described, they testified that the lack of understanding of the particular nuances that ASC brings to a relationship meant that they were often treated in an unsatisfactory manner.

A Double-Edged Sword

Rather than improving the situation, the course of action taken by most service providers, frequently exacerbated their distress while leaving them with little option for other appropriate assistance.

FIONA

But what I found in the situation of going to counsellors or psychologists for the both of us, he comes over sounding very polished and very academic and I show up as being this emotional wreck ... Well, we went to a behavioural psychologist. That's when it really started going downhill, and she was telling William to do things like you would an ordinary couple, a married couple who are having problems and she was telling him to do things that he couldn't have done in a million years. And that's when the real conflict started ... Yeah so, I can see the damage that the wrong psychologist can do.

KATY

I have had some very humiliating experiences with doctors where they immediately take his side and if I have anything to say, I am just being overbearing, and they see me as the problem, and they see it as a marital problem, and so they recommend having marital counselling ... It's rare that you find a counsellor that really understands ... I find that devastating because it is so contrary to the person that I am and I am suddenly depicted as this overbearing, dragon of a person, simply because, um, I don't know why. Because they don't see the dynamic.

Have We Gone Nuts?

SOPHIE   *Other than tons of self-help books, university courses in communication; not involving AS, and the occasional discussion with my mother, no. In the United States, mental health care and counselling are expensive even when covered by insurance. For most, counselling is a luxury. I personally cannot afford this service.*

LUCY   *A psychologist is very expensive too. One trained in Asperger is very expensive, I've spent my hard earned, and he doesn't seem to appreciate that, just to keep me. Recently, because I just walked away from him a couple of months ago, I said, 'Look this is what I needed to do. I need you to go and learn strategies', and I've got to do the same thing because it's like speaking in a different language. I'll still be doing the heavy lifting as far as I can see but ... 'I need you to please go to this psychologist and be assessed and learn some strategies and then I'll be right there with you.' So, the next minute he rings me up and says, 'Oh well I contacted the psychologist.' I said, 'Oh okay, I'm really proud of you', and then I thought, 'Are you just spinning me a line?' But no, he sent me the email that they'd sent him back, and here we go again he can be so generous on one hand and so mean on the other. So, when I went to see him about it, I said 'You're not going to go are you?' He said, 'Too much money', and he had just got a bonus and I said, 'Do you realise that I've*

224

already spent that amount of money on finding out about this?' That part just went straight over his head. He didn't care that I earn half his wages, yet I had spent this money ... and I said to him, 'I think the relationship is worth it but clearly you don't.'

MANDY   *There's not a lot of places for adults, and groups to go and sort through problems and I think one on one would probably be better, but again it's time and money and all the other things that go with seeking professional help ... at the moment we've just been doing it together.*

BETH   *We went to Relationships Australia and basically the counsellor pulled me aside and said you have to leave him. Yeah, she was trying to get me to leave him, but I could see a glimmer, you know. I could see he was a good person. Yeah, but then I started to see a psychologist and she's very positive, yeah, yep.*

Whereas Dianne (NT) believed that Jim's (ASC) lack of engagement with therapy was why it had failed for them:

So yes, we have had lots of other services, but they really haven't made any difference. Even ... recently doing that Relationship Minefields with the Minds and Hearts. He would come home and say, 'Yeah it was all right', but the wives all were asked at the last night, and then most of us found out they had had work to do. It was an 8-week thing, but they had had work to do every week that they hadn't even come home and shared. We didn't even know that they had homework. There were things that they were supposed to do with us, but most of them hadn't done it. You know, and it was like I just said to him, 'Why would you spend all this money and do this stuff and not do...'. 'Oooh, because if I did – you would've...'. See the same. So not willing to step out of their comfort zone and have a go.

Each to Their Own

Since the neurotypical world often has different expectations for communication and social behaviour, it is usually hard for adults with ASC to navigate support systems designed with neurotypical communication styles in mind. Georgia (NT) said that while counselling had helped her, she wondered if it was the same for those on the spectrum:

One of the big things I did was to say, 'I'm not dealing this very well so I need to go find out what I need to do to deal with it better', and that's when I went into counselling and it was a slow process but you start to spiral upwards and outwards instead of spiralling down and just taking steps back, then you find these forums and you think, do Asperger people have similar sort of support groups because I mean they must feel pain. They must feel rejection. They feel like misfits. They feel like nobody understands them. Do they have similar types of forums and support groups and within the forums and support groups are they encouraged to try and adapt or modify their behaviour so they can work with neurotypicals or are they encouraged to well you are who you are, so you know be strong, be empowered and be proud to be different.

A Double-Edged Sword

William (ASC) said that seeking support from groups did not really work for him:

In the groups I find that they don't really work, because the thing about Asperger's is you're too fearful of speaking up in a group, and so that's what it results in. Especially about bad experiences earlier, and that's one of my special problems. But 26 years in the public service has given me some skills in speaking in meetings and such like. I can actually do it without dying inside quite as much, but that's a degree of control which is only good for formal situations. You can't begin to speak in another group at your own personal level. Some can, I suppose, and they do. I went to one group, and I didn't say a word, I don't think. I just listened to the rest, so it didn't do me any good.

Given that people with ASC experience difficulties with verbal and nonverbal communication, expressing their needs and feelings, and understanding the responses or advice they receive, they often prefer to seek help in different ways to neurotypicals. One way is through online forums. These forums are online discussion sites where people can hold conversations in the form of posted messages and are much better suited to communication styles of people on the spectrum. Not only do they provide an online exchange of information between people about a particular topic, but they are also a valuable resource to connect, share experiences and seek support.

In her conversation, Georgia (NT) sought to understand what happens in the online forums for those with ASC. When mentioning that one of the topics covered was the perception that the NT population feels a considerable amount of anger towards them, she replied:

Have We Gone Nuts?

So, what you experience in your close intimate relationship is basically what they carry into their forums ... Well, that's interesting, I don't know about you, but that's something that my husband says to me, and when you say to them, 'I'm not angry. I'm frustrated because I don't seem to be able to get you to understand me and it's important for me to have you understand me.'

She went on to say:

I've read some books looking at what Asperger's guys have said ... 'even if you don't understand why you're doing it just do it because it helps your partner'. And this is what [that] David Finch guy said, 'I don't always understand why I'm doing it, but I know it's the right thing to do and it makes ... things good in our family and ... I want to make things good in our family' ... I just thought it was good, it helped me believe that I think Aspie people can adapt if they want to, but they have to want to.

In contrast to ASC participants, most NT participants found that face-to-face support groups or support groups online were 'a lifesaver' that provided much needed answers. Dawn said as much:

All of this has been helped HUGELY by learning more and more about autism and being able to finally put two and two together and finding that forum, who's been a lifesaver for me, really has ... I can't remember if I told you that, that was how I worked it out ... I came across, I think it was a DT forum, or the website initially, and ... they have a bit that has anecdotes by people who have gone through it, about how it made them feel and ... it was that that made me realise, it wasn't his behaviour, it was the NTs saying how they felt and I began to think 'that's how I feel'.

Tracy said that support groups and forums have been 'invaluable' to her:

What has been most helpful have been support groups online. I am a member of one such group though they are in Australia, and I am in France. We write regularly back and forth and share news. I also participate in two forums, an English one and a German one. It has been invaluable.

Similarly, Nora found that the understanding obtained from support groups and online forums to be reassuring:

I've got the support group and online forum so I'm only really willing to talk to people that know about Asperger's or are in a similar situation because they just 'get it' and there's no need to kind of explain it too much, and there's no grey areas. When you talk to somebody who lives with an Asperger's person, they totally are onto it, they totally get it. You're understood. You feel like you've had a chat. You feel like you've gotten something off your chest. You've had a good laugh because it is bloody funny sometimes and that's it.

Quinn mentioned that she had found the information about this research through her support group:

I do have one and that's how I learned about your research and those ladies have been very, very helpful, but it has been very helpful to be in that group. Yeah, I love my support groups, if it wasn't for that ... yeah, and there's a lot of ladies from Australia too and that side of the world. So, that's nice because when you're crying and writing something at midnight, there's always somebody there that will see it and answer.

Looking for Silver Linings

Due to ongoing disappointments from being let down by service providers and the friends and family members who were more often a source of negativity than support, the majority of ASC and NT participants were compelled to turn to other resources to find answers. As the participants' mentioned, they were often able to locate positive sources of information, solutions and much needed understanding through online forums, face-to-face or online support groups, and these support opportunities provided the silver lining in the midst of the frequent negativity they encountered. However, while these were constructive avenues of support, these support sources were mainly independent of each other, providing encouragement in individually autistic or individually NT settings. Understanding that there is the need for appropriate support sources that work equally in cooperation with each other for both is essential for developing targeted supports and interventions, for those with autism and their partners and family members. Georgia (NT) looked towards the potential for a more positive future:

Yeah, and like you say these support groups and knowledge and information and reading and learning and you know, the support and just validation and knowing that you're not alone and knowing that there's people, it's almost like people are coming out of the woodwork now you know. It's kind of like the stigma that was attached to mental illness and people wouldn't talk about it or being gay and people wouldn't talk about it, now it's like, 'Oh people are listening. There are a few that are listening, and then now more are listening, and you keep growing that population of people who have suffered and then the voice gets louder and then people start to listen.

Support Thoughts

Neurodiverse relationships may possibly be regarded as intercultural relationships in some respects, yet with their own unique challenges as well as producing opportunities for growth. The study by Smith et al. (2020) found that people in these relationships were more likely to succeed when they were able to develop an array of personalised strategies that allowed them to work together through the conflict created by their unconventional communication skills and patterns. Furthermore, although they confirmed in their study that the NT participants played a significant role in assisting the autistic person in social interactions, the most significant finding of the study was how the possibilities for doing well increased when each person was willing to continuously adapt to increase the potential to work together through their inevitable challenges (Smith et al., 2020).

However, usually doing well is made possible when having the opportunity to find appropriate assistance. Since a low level of expertise with autism is a contributing factor to the overall treatment dissatisfaction for people with ASC (Lipinski et al., 2019) and a lack of education and knowledge plays a major role in therapists' willingness to accept autistic adults for treatment (Lipinski et al., 2021), it goes without saying that the need for an increase in knowledge and understanding about autism in adulthood is essential.

In the next chapter, the participants provide their knowledge, expertise and guidance to aid in the general understanding and assessment of people in neurodiverse relationships.

11

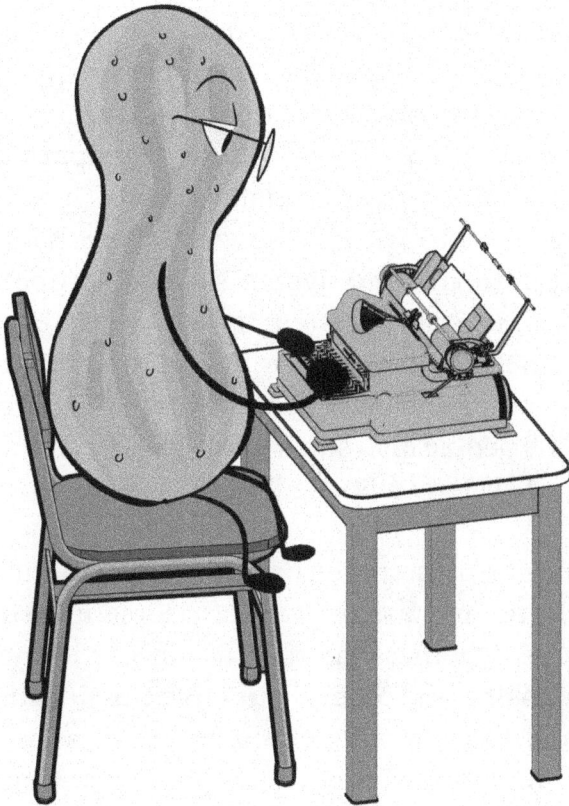

Seeking an Urgent Upgrade

Have We Gone Nuts?

'Sometimes the loudest cries for help are silent.'
Harlan Coben

The pairing of ASC and NT people appears to produce notably similar relationships regardless of the significant variability within each group and between each group. Consequently, it is important to recognise that when a relationship includes both autistic and neurotypical people, regardless of the distinct individualities of each person, their relationship will most likely follow a comparable pattern to most other neurodiverse relationships. This comparable pattern appears to include several remarkably similar additional patterns and systems. Book 1 reports on the specific communication system the appears to be a common occurrence in these relationships. As reported throughout this book, many other unconventional relational aspects between ASC and NT people also seem to evolve into many different patterns and systems between them.

Looking for these patterns and systems will aid in the understanding and assessment of people in neurodiverse relationships, whether classified as similar to intercultural relationships or some other distinctive classification. Due to the blend of two differently wired brains, these relationships may be viewed as complex systems, all operating similarly. Identification of the many common unconventional features unique to these relationships will foster an ability to better provide appropriate treatment and interventions.

Chalk and Cheese

It is important for service providers, friends and family members of those in neurodiverse relationships, together with people in these relationships, to become familiar with the differences that set these relationships apart from conventional relationships. The following paragraph summarises the main factors that contribute to the unconventionality of neurodiverse relationships described in detail throughout this book.

Regardless of their differences, all people with ASC are characterised primarily by early-onset difficulties in reciprocal social behaviour. Neurotypical people, tend to have instinctive reciprocal social and emotional skills. Autism impacts on the way a person understands, communicates with and relates to others and the world around them. Neurotypical people do not display autistic or other neurologically atypical patterns of thought, communication or behaviour. Autistic people place less emphasis on social interactions in preference for non-social activities. Neurotypical people place more emphasis on having many opportunities to communicate, connect, express love and give and receive emotional support. Specific features within these main factors are:

Social Communication

Neurotypical: Typically engages in social interactions easily, understands and uses nonverbal cues (facial expressions, body language, tone of voice) effectively, and easily develops and maintains relationships.

Autistic: May have challenges with social communication, including difficulties with nonverbal cues, understanding social norms and maintaining eye contact. Some individuals with autism may struggle with reciprocal conversations.

Repetitive Behaviours and Interests

Neurotypical: Displays a range of interests and behaviours, but typically not to the same intensity, single-mindedness or restricted focus as seen in autism. May have preferences or routines, but these are usually held less rigidly than seen in autism.

Autistic: Often engages in repetitive behaviours or has intense interests that are more limited in scope. These behaviours or interests can be a source of comfort and may help regulate sensory experiences.

Sensory Sensitivities

Neurotypical: Generally, tolerates a wide range of sensory stimuli without significant distress.

Autistic: May experience heightened sensitivities or hypo-sensitivities to sensory stimuli (e.g. lights, sounds, textures). This can impact the individual's comfort and functioning in various environments.

Communication Challenges

Neurotypical: Typically develops language skills in a typical sequence and uses language for a variety of communicative functions.

Autistic: Language development may be delayed or atypical. Some individuals may have difficulties with expressive or receptive language skills. Communication challenges can vary widely, from nonverbal to highly articulate.

Flexibility and Routine

Neurotypical: Generally adaptable to changes in routine or plans.

Autistic: Often prefers routine and may experience distress when routines are disrupted. A need for sameness and resistance to change is common.

Theory of Mind

Neurotypical: Typically understands and is aware of others' perspectives, thoughts and emotions.

Autistic: May have challenges with theory of mind, which involves understanding that others can have different beliefs, intentions and emotions. This can impact social interactions and empathy.

While it is crucial to emphasise that autism is a spectrum, and individuals with autism can have a wide range of strengths and challenges, the above points condense the information provided by Book 1 and also throughout this book.

Additionally, the concept of neurotypicality is a generalisation and doesn't capture the diversity of neurotypical individuals. Every person is unique, and these generalisations should not be applied rigidly to any individual. However, these generalisations will aid in appreciating the many unconventional aspects of neurodiverse relationships since it is the pairing of different neurologies that cultivate a different type of relationship.

It is important to note that, often, autistic adults do not present in public as autistic due to their notable skills in camouflaging their traits. Often, neurotypical adults present as physically and emotionally overwrought in public, with an appearance of mental health challenges and chronic health issues due to managing the non-standard behaviour of their ASC partners and family members. These matters require appropriate understanding and different techniques than standard therapies and treatments to support all people in neurodiverse relationships.

Words from the Wise

Interview participants were asked questions regarding their viewpoints and thoughts or ideas on options that they would like to see happen. Participants with ASC mostly hoped for more education and awareness:

RACHELLE *It would be just so much better if local doctors picked up on it more ... Sort of say, 'Hang on. There's something funny going on here. This person might be on the spectrum', and that's the start of getting help, because I've been floating around the system for thirty-five years and it wasn't picked up.*

MARK *It is more that there is a general awareness ... You look at what's been done over the last few years, say with some of the depression initiatives 'Beyond Blue' and that sort of ... information at doctors' surgeries ... They now talk about in high schools and having that general awareness of mental health issues. I think it would be very beneficial ... if there was an awareness ... in high school or primary school, science classes, more information in the curriculum about ... the human condition, that is, that people are aware ... of differences.*

RICHARD *I suppose more awareness ... When you tell somebody, you've got Asperger's Syndrome, a lot of people, it just goes right over their head, and they've got no real understanding of what it's really about ... but as I say what you're doing and the more information that we can sort of channel it's all going to help in the end.*

SAMUEL *Acceptance of the differences ... so that people understand when a person with Asperger's responds in what they would consider inappropriate, instead of just dismissing it outright, taking the time to hear it out a bit further.*

STELLA *More understanding and acceptance, especially for women on the spectrum.*

TERRY *I think education would be one thing so that people can be aware that there are these differences ... and it's generally not a conscious choice to be that way and there are differences in the brain and the way we operate that actually make us who we are and make us different.*

Have We Gone Nuts?

When asked how we can achieve the potential for more education and awareness, Max said:

I think people do actually change when they realise that's the way things are done and sometimes that change doesn't accrue overnight, like for instance, we want change so that people don't drink and drive ... Years ago, if you got busted drink driving, your friends will say to you, 'Oh that's a shame. That's bad luck' ... Now if you get caught drink driving your friends give you a ribbing, 'You dickhead! Why do you drink and drive, you moron' ... I think that when people start feeling like that's just the way things are done, that's when change happens.

Some ASC participants also shared their ideas on how to make change happen in their relationships:

BARRY   *Couples sitting together saying, 'Have you found this, have you found that?'... You might have them sitting in a circle ... I suppose like alcoholics anonymous ... I just think that would be an approach ... small groups like that ... It certainly would help people to realise that they are not the only ones having a problem and it is a solvable problem.*

TOM   *Some kind of online exercise or game that builds relationship skills would be nice. Thank you for including me in this project. As an older adult on the spectrum, I feel ignored by most autism professionals and organisations.*

MURRAY   *The Asperger's person needs to make sure that they're putting the full effort in and not using it as a cop out and I think the non-Asperger person needs to understand that there's certain elements of the personality you're not going to change ... That things relating to Asperger's that he's doing, he's not doing to hurt you, he's doing it because that's the way he is. I think understanding on their part versus more effort on the Asperger's part are probably the key.*

Most NT participants shared similar views about education and awareness and various ideas they had for support, interventions and also to introduce change:

MIA   *I think awareness is a huge issue, awareness amongst professionals in terms of the GPs, psychiatrists and psychologists, awareness is massive. I'd like to see support for the neurotypical partners, but a support that is positive and encouraging ... so I'd like to see awareness, I'd like to see a more positive approach to dealing with these relationships.*

RENEE   *What I'd like to happen is that there would be much more awareness in the community, in the marriage guidance whatever they call themselves, relationship services ... most of us have been through heaps of counsellors who have never seen anything like this and so that does more damage than no counselling whatsoever.*

BETH   *I think more community awareness, like with typical behaviours of an AS person ... they could do television ads, I don't know, or some advertisements ... 'Are you feeling anxious? Could your partner be on the spectrum, does he/she do this?'*

DAWN   *I think increasing awareness all the time ... I think the internet is such a phenomenal way of disseminating information ... to communicate personal experience to people is how you get them to understand. I have known about Temple Grandin for probably 10 years. I've read some of what she has done, I've watched some of her, what she has done, I still didn't make the connection. Now she, to me is what autism is. The internet is such an amazing form of communication. I think webinars ... and podcasts and using or communicating through the better-quality radio and TV resources, whether it's the BBC or the Australian version or the US version ... using any medium, media to disseminate the information, the personal experience, so that is going to help the spouses ... I think ... training more and more specialists who truly understand autism and how it can affect the person and their relationships and people who are on the receiving end of their personalities. I don't know if, as we come to a better understanding, we can help ... so I mean and that's all down to funding isn't it, so how do you get the funding to keep training more people and keep this study going.*

WINNIE   *More research would be helpful. I think perhaps more education ... right back to ... the universities who are counselling some psychology students, social workers, medical students. ... when I go to groups and see women ... I hear their stories of their reception from certain counsellors, or just the general community of, lack of understanding and I just think 'There is so much more that needs to be done and more ways to go' ... of being believed, understood, accepted for what's happening to them.*

KAY   *More local support programs ... I would like to be able to see intervention programs. You know and tools and of which there are none ... That's what I need ... And we need funding because we have missed the child cut off and now, they know more about it ... So not only are we costing the taxpayer money you know with health, but it could be assisted financially not only from the government, but we could take less from the government if we had funding for things, we could do ourselves. To me it's a cost benefit ... I'm sure we would be costing the government less from accessing some of the services. So, I think it's a worthwhile thing that you are doing. Those tools are essential. Intervention is essential then it doesn't have to be a clinical psych intervention … You have obviously hit upon something that is so needed for people. That's good. It's remarkable, isn't it? How you started out. And how you stumbled across … It's unfolding. It's incredible. Yeah. It's opening up broader.*

WANDA *A communication tool. How's that! A training package … for our relationships.*

HOLLY *I think awareness. A lot of it would be around knowledge and understanding from others, but I think some really good clear books on how to work through problems.*

SOPHIE *Having access, as well as plenty of professional therapists and counsellors knowledgeable in ASD would be a blessing.*

QUINN *It would be nice to have a better knowledge of maybe how the NT person can communicate with the AS person to get to connect somehow in a level that they can connect, because I feel that there has to be a way. We just don't have the tools. It's like speaking different languages.*

LUCY *I think it's got to be more widely understood. It's probably one of the least understood things out there … and that's why I say [the program] Insight because they're so compassionate with the way they deal with things … How do you get people believing it because if they just look up Dr Google, they get 30 questions and in the Asperger's mind, like [my partner] thinks he's very social.*

RAE *If there was some sort of tool that we could, even if it was all on video, we could bring it home, couldn't we? Like a DVD, a role-play, and you could have like 20 conversations just around the kitchen.*

KATY *Sometimes I almost feel that it would be good to have a permanent mediator that can just sit, hear both sides of the story ... A translator. Someone to interpret for me, but also to be able to interpret for him ... If you had, for instance, a support group where something like that was developed and ... have someone that can actually use both kinds of language ... The thing that kills me is the fact that it is a close personal relationship, where it becomes impossible.*

DIANNE *A buddy system or something. You have another couple in the same situation, and the blokes talk to one another about how they deal with this and the females. I have no idea whether that would work or not ... Mentors maybe ... supporting, mentoring ... so we improve ... become more aware. How can we best support people who are in the same situation ... and maybe you could even, have an education and training group.*

Have We Gone Nuts?

HALEY   *I would really, really like to see that if this study can do it, is to show, or to be able to teach ways of … just so that you can have a normal conversation without it blowing up. Or … just to have as normal a relationship … just to be able to talk normally, not to have to think about every word that you say because it is all going to be taken so literally.*

HAZEL   *People with Asperger usually have a special interest, or a vocation that they are so good at, but they end up doing measly, menial jobs like packing shelves or carting boxes or warehouse stuff … beneath their intellectual… and so if there was a service where people with Asperger…could go to a…employment service thing and where … [they] did not go for an interview.*

RYAN   *For the future … I think the more people who are diagnosed and are out about it. I mean … if people with ASD are open about it and out about it, they'd help a hell of a lot. The more people that you have in your life saying, 'Well I'm on the spectrum' …it's going to be a great win … I think it's much better with openness.*

Support Thoughts

It is crucial for service providers and practitioners, friends and family members of those in neurodiverse relationships, as well as policy makers and other stakeholders to listen to the words of the participants. Their words will inform ways to craft avenues for support, program improvement and future program development. Additionally, academics should consider the findings, presented through the words of the participants, in creating new, or refining existing, interventions and programs for people in neurodiverse relationships as it directly incorporates their voices. Consideration for the findings of these studies, as they align with existing research on the lack of service needs of adults with ASC, such as Koffer Miller et al. (2018), Zerbo et al. (2015), Warfield et al. (2015), together with the needs of their partners and family members, should be at the forefront in designing and improving services and supports that meet the unique needs of this population.

In the final chapter, the key messages of the book are revealed as we summarise the unconventionality of neurodiverse relationships and look forward to a time when the unknown aspects of adult autism and their relationships become more known.

12

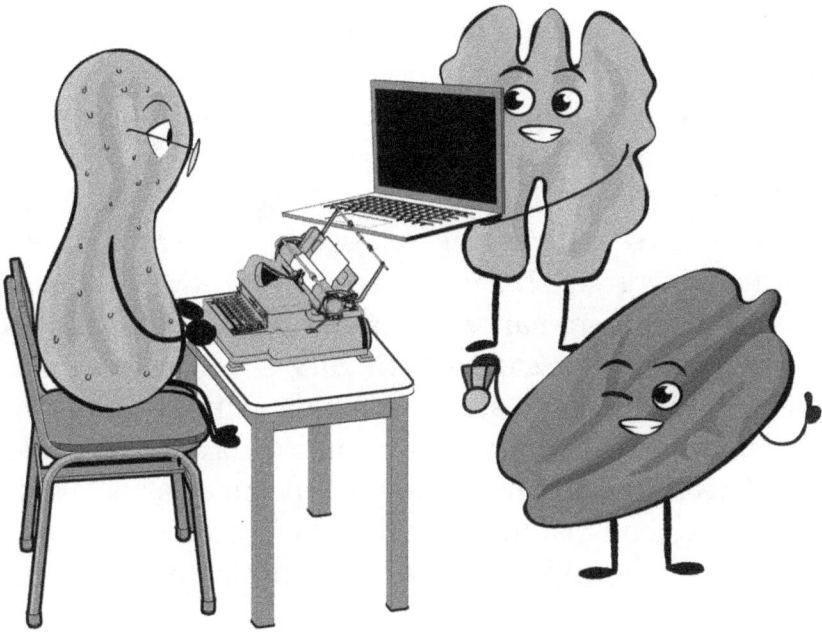

Steps Forward

Have We Gone Nuts?

'So, let us not be blind to our differences – but let us also direct attention to our common interests and to the means by which those differences can be resolved.'
John F. Kennedy

Research has established that conventional healthy relationships share specific patterns including open communication, shared experiences, honesty, trust and mutual respect. There is no imbalance of power. Each other's independence is respected. Each can make their own decisions without fear of retribution or retaliation, and each share decisions. These patterns make it possible to build a life together that has a sense of shared purpose and meaning, lifelong companionship, romance, support, sexual fulfillment and commitment (Ariyo & Mgbeokwii, 2019; Gottman & Gottman, 2017). However, Ariyo and Mgbeokwii (2019) state that 'the greater the gap between two people in terms of attitudes, values, habits, recreational activities and temperaments, the greater is the likelihood that they will find themselves incompatible and unable to form [a] workable relationship' (p. 1).

Whether or not they actually do develop over time, generally people expect their relationships will include these healthy relationship patterns. However, neurodiverse relationships do not correspond to conventional patterns. Due to the combination of two different neurologies, neurodiverse relationships take on unconventional qualities that are not only similar to Ariyo and Mgbeokwii's description of an incompatible relationship, but these incompatibilities usually only become known to those inside the relationship. Often, others get the impression that these relationships are conventional, reasonably healthy relationships.

Fundamentals of Change

Education about neurodiverse relationships is a vital step toward creating a more inclusive and understanding society. By promoting awareness, challenging stereotypes and fostering empathy, we can contribute to building stronger, more supportive communities for everyone, regardless of neurodivergent traits. Here are some strategies for education and for developing your understanding that can be beneficial for people in neurodiverse relationships:

Education and Understanding: Both should invest time in learning about each other's neurotypes. Understanding the differences and similarities in thinking, communication and behaviour is crucial. Education can help reduce misunderstandings and promote empathy.

Effective Communication: Working towards developing strong communication skills is essential. Both should allow each other to openly discuss their needs, boundaries and preferences. Using clear and direct language, allowing processing time and allowing time for communicating the whole message can help prevent misinterpretations.

Empathy and Patience: Both should practise empathy and patience and appreciate each other's differences. People with ASC have different sensory sensitivities or communication styles, which can require a more patient and understanding response from others. People who are NT might need more time to talk through their thoughts in order to feel heard.

Flexible Problem-Solving: Finding solutions to challenges may require creativity and flexibility. It's important to find ways to work together to adapt and find approaches that work for both.

Social Skills Training: For people with ASC who struggle with social skills, social skills training can be beneficial. Allowing the NT people in your life to become your social secretaries can support learning to better know how to navigate social situations and understand social cues. This learning can improve interactions within all relationships.

Respect for Autonomy: Both should respect each other's autonomy and individuality. It's essential to strike a balance between spending quality time together and allowing each other space for personal interests and activities.

Advocacy and Accommodations: Neurotypical people can play a vital role in advocating for their partners and family members with ASC when it comes to accommodations at work or in other aspects of life. Accommodations can significantly improve the quality of life for those with autism.

Here are some additional key points to consider when educating others about neurodiverse relationships:

Diverse Perspectives: Neurodiverse relationships often involve people with different cognitive styles, communication preferences and sensory sensitivities. Growing an understanding and appreciation of these differences can lead to richer, more diverse perspectives within relationships.

Communication Challenges: People in neurodiverse relationships may experience challenges in communication and social interaction. It's essential to educate others about alternative communication methods, such as visual supports, social stories and clear verbal communication, to facilitate effective interaction.

Embracing Differences: Rather than viewing neurodiversity as a hindrance, it's important to embrace the unique strengths and abilities that each bring to a relationship. This may include a heightened attention to detail versus big picture thinking, creativity or a different way of problem-solving.

Reducing Stigma: Education can help break down stigmas associated with neurodivergence. By promoting awareness and understanding, we can challenge stereotypes and misconceptions, fostering an environment of acceptance and support.

Supporting Inclusivity: Neurodiverse relationships may require accommodations and adjustments to create inclusive spaces. By educating those around us, we can advocate for and implement inclusive practices in various settings, including schools, workplaces and social events.

Empathy and Patience: Building empathy is crucial in neurodiverse relationships. Understanding that each experiences the world differently to the other and each has unique needs to the other requires patience, flexibility and a willingness to adapt.

Advocacy and Allyship: Educating ourselves enables us to become advocates and allies for ourselves and others in similar relationships. This involves challenging discriminatory practices, promoting inclusive policies and amplifying the voices of those in neurodiverse communities.

Relationship Dynamics: Neurodiverse relationships have unique dynamics, and it's important to recognise and respect these differences. By understanding each person's needs and preferences, we can create healthier and more supportive relationships.

Making Headway

Once those in neurodiverse relationships are aware of the reasons underpinning their incompatibilities, it becomes possible to begin the journey towards understanding and forming a workable relationship. Educating ourselves and attempting to educate others about the unconventionality of neurodiverse relationships is crucial for growing and adapting in our relationships and also fostering understanding, empathy and inclusivity in our communities. Winnie (NT) described how her growing understanding of autism blossomed into helping others to understand:

> *That couples' counsellor that I saw has other clients and so … it dawned on me over some long period of time … what my husband had was ASD and so I gradually brought it up with the counsellor and it was over some time that they became convinced, and I showed, I talked about articles, I talked about what was said at the groups, not about individuals, and then compared them with him, so it was sort of, in a way, I was educating the counsellor. I have no clear memory of how I got onto Asperger's but the more I read about it, and then I got books from the library written by women who were in marriages and then I went online and I think the common story too, we will just read everything that is available because here is something that sounds exactly like what is happening in my*

*life and I've never heard of it, don't know anything about it.
I want to know everything because it is explaining my life ...
It was just like 'Oh my God! There're other people out there',
and so then I showed her the book that I got from the library
and talked about what they said, and so with all of that, she
started saying 'Oh well, I've got these clients and this is what
the husband's saying,' and I'm saying 'Well', and then the
more she worked with them the more she realised that that
husband was on the spectrum and so she got more clients like
that that made her understand and they came to see her ...
They always seem to be the older men, so it's that undiagnosed
group that didn't have anything when they were children ...
that's another awareness I would be out of the league of if I
hadn't gone to support groups ... From what the women that I
have read about, the women that I have met in the group, I am
just amazed by (a) their resilience and (b) persistence too and
the hard work they put in to learn and you know the efforts
to make the relationship work and to teach themselves about
the condition rather than just walk away ... and that was the
turning point for me, because I was reaching a point where
I wanted to walk away, but it's having that understanding
that it's not a maliciousness, or you know a willful intent to
cause any distress, but it just they are struggling, you know
with living their lives the best way they can.*

Some participants expressed gratitude about their
involvement in the studies. Georgia (NT) said:

*And the thing is, you're helping, and you will help and the
outcome of your research and what you find is going to
help so many people. Yeah, I mean if these communication
issues are really identified and seen that they can have such
devastating effects on couples, you can start at a much earlier*

stage when you identify Asperger's in a child you can start those therapies, those treatments to help them to exist in a relationship in a healthy way. It will just make so much difference to people's lives.

Similarly, Wally (ASC) said:

I thank you for the opportunity to talk. I think the kind of questions that you're asking are the kind of questions that I would like my psychologist to ask of the both of us. I think that there are a number of things that you're asking which are not the sort of standard marriage guidance type ... There's stuff there that I'd like my partner to hear that I don't think you can say as part of an ordinary couple's conversation. You know there are a couple of things there you said, 'Well do you think you could say this to your partner?' Well, the context of our conversation was very, very different and to find the right time to say something like those is very hard. On the other hand, for NT partners and Aspie partners to read perhaps some of the things that your interviewees are saying is probably going to be valuable. To be honest a lot of the stuff out there in books and so forth about these types of relationships is not positive at all ... so if you can find ways of putting some of the point of view of, I'm assuming that most of the Aspie spouses that you're talking to actually do care as much as I do, so put that over right ... And it's not a matter of not knowing how, you see you can learn scripts, you can write lists you can do all this stuff, and maybe that's part of the not believing that you were getting at before. So what you have to say, that you have to pay attention more, that you have to learn how to do this active listening, so why isn't it happening? Why is it impossible to do? It's not that I don't want to. Wanda will say 'There's things that you forget.'

The little things that she's told you, that amongst everything else that you've forgotten, that's she's going out on Saturday afternoon, you've forgotten it, so therefore it's not important to you. No, it's not correct. And it's the same with the things that you have to try and do to make it work. Firstly, when you're in that moment of anxiety all the scripts are gone. All the step-by-step processes that you're supposed to be able to draw on through your cognitive behaviour therapy all that stuff when it comes down to it in that moment, the lack of emotional control, the lack of ability to connect your head and your heart together. No. Before I was diagnosed, I was having some problems and I went to see a counsellor and she said, 'I've never met somebody so disconnected between their head and their heart as you.' Because I could be in a blubbering mess and then give her a cognitive description of what was going on in my mind and just switch between those things. But when you're in that state, when you're in that moment of not knowing how to deal with something, being blindsided by something, all the CBT processes in the world aren't going to help you.

In a Nutshell

The lack of community understanding of autism has had quite a significant negative impact on people with autism and on their partners and family members. It has contributed to misconceptions and stigmas surrounding autism. It has often led to judgemental attitudes, a lack of tolerance and a lack of support from friends and family, professionals who work with this population and even within the broader community. Sabrina (NT), stated the viewpoint of the majority of both ASC and NT participants:

Have We Gone Nuts?

Since so many of these relationship issues naturally end up in marriage counselling ... there needs to be a better job done in the education of psychologists, social workers ... so that they don't inflict the traditional counselling on [them] ... It's never going to work, and it's just going to cause more harm than good.

In communities where there is limited awareness of autism, there may be a scarcity of resources and support services for individuals and couples dealing with neurodiversity. This lack of infrastructure can make it challenging for people in neurodiverse relationships to access the help and guidance they may need. It may also make it very expensive to access any limited resources and support services that there may be.

If the community does not understand or appreciate the specific differences and difficulties that develop in a relationship from the unique communication styles of those with ASC it can trigger misinterpretations, frustration and a lack of empathy. As a result, it can make it difficult for people in neurodiverse relationships to navigate social situations and can put a strain on relationships.

Societal expectations around social norms and relationship dynamics can be particularly challenging for neurodiverse couples and families. The lack of understanding often leads people on the autism spectrum to feel pressured to conform to neurotypical expectations, potentially causing them much stress and anxiety. Likewise, NT individuals often feel pressured to conceal the reality of their lives, potentially causing them much stress and anxiety. Consequently, this lack of understanding of autism means that the majority of people in neurodiverse relationships are left feeling isolated without any ability to reach out for appropriate understanding and support.

To address these issues, it's essential to promote education and awareness about autism within communities. Increased community understanding can play a crucial role in promoting acceptance and empathy. Educational initiatives that aim to raise awareness about autism, its strengths, and challenges, can contribute to a more inclusive and supportive environment. Communities that actively work towards inclusivity and acceptance of neurodiversity provide a more positive environment for individuals in neurodiverse relationships. This includes fostering open conversations, organising events that promote awareness, and creating spaces where everyone feels welcome. This can lead to increased acceptance, reduced stigma and better support networks for individuals in neurodiverse relationships. Additionally, fostering a culture of empathy and understanding can contribute to creating a more inclusive and supportive community for everyone. Daniel (ASC) shared his hope for the future:

As our autistic children move into adulthood, drawing back the veil on adult autism would be an appropriate gift to them.

Final Thoughts

While there is still much to learn about neurodiverse relationships, the findings of the two studies highlight participants' perspectives concerning what takes place when they reach out to others to access support and/ or services. The aim of this book is to present these findings through the words of the 400 participants in order to improve understanding of their reality. Listening to the voices of those in neurodiverse relationships, not only contributes valuable insights into their lived experience but also gives others an understanding of how to provide comfort and support to them. By improving understanding of their unique experiences, opportunities are provided to work towards finding solutions to overcome the effects of the lack of professional and community knowledge about adult autism and the resulting impacts on relationships, and on their abilities to access appropriate professional help.

Findings also stress the need for greater community awareness and education about issues confronting those in neurodiverse relationships to reduce the distress felt by these families. It is hoped that through hearing from the participants in these studies, it will promote greater understanding and aid in bridging the knowledge gap that currently exists between many service providers, the community in general, and the unique relationship experiences of neurodiverse families and couples.

The third book of the *Have They Gone Nuts?* series shares the research data. The graphs and tables illustrate similarities and differences between the two groups of people and also gives valuable insights into male/female similarities and differences. It will be crucial for policy makers, practitioners and other stakeholders to utilise the data from this study to inform program improvement and future program development. Academics should consider the data gained from this study in crafting new, or refining existing, research, interventions and programs for people in neurodiverse relationships as it directly incorporates their voices. Look out for this next book in the series to further enhance your understanding of the neurodiverse experience from the inside.

References

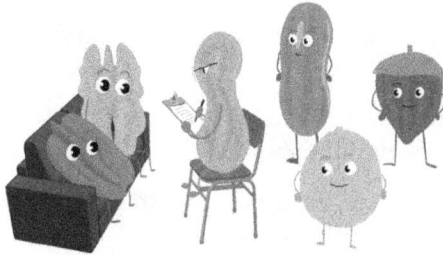

Anon. (2020). Raising awareness of the impact of autism in long-term intimate adult relationships in Australia. Select Committee on Autism.

Arad, P. (2020). *When your man is on the spectrum: To know, understand and transform your relationship.* Independently published.

Arad, P., Shechtman, Z., & Attwood, T. (2022). Physical and mental well-being of women in neurodiverse relationships: A comparative study. *Journal of Psychology & Psychotherapy, 12*(1), 1-9.

Arioli, M., Crespi, C., & Canessa, N. (2018). Social cognition through the lens of cognitive and clinical neuroscience. *BioMed Research International, 2018,* 4283427. https://doi.org/10.1155/2018/4283427

Ariyo, A. M., & Mgbeokwii, G. N. (2019). Perception of companionship in relation to marital satisfaction : a study of married men and women. *IFE PsychologIA : An International Journal, 27*(1), 1-8.

Arora, T. (2012). Understanding the perseveration displayed by students with Autism Spectrum Disorder. *Education, 132*(4), 799-808. https://doi.org/10.1016/j.rasd.2011.01.003

Aston, M. (2003a). Asperger Syndrome in the Counselling Room. *Counselling and Psychotherapy Journal, 14*(5), 10-13. www.maxineaston. co.uk

Aston, M. (2003b). *Aspergers in love. Couple relationships and family affairs.* Jessica Kingsley Publishers.

Atherton, G., Edisbury, E., Piovesan, A., & Cross, L. (2021). Autism through the ages: A mixed methods approach to understanding how age and age of diagnosis affect quality of life. *Journal of Autism and Developmental Disorders*, 1-16.

Attwood, T. (2007). *The complete guide to Asperger's Syndrome.* Jessica Kingsley Publishers.

Attwood, T. (2015). *The complete guide to Asperger's Syndrome* (Revised ed.). Jessica Kingsley Publishers.

Attwood, T., Evans, C. R., & Lesko, A. (2014). *Been there. Done that. Try this!* Jessica Kingsley Publishers.

Baez, S., & Ibanez, A. (2014). The effects of context processing on social cognition impairments in adults with Asperger's syndrome. *Frontiers in Neuroscience, 8*(270), 1-9. https://doi.org/10.3389/fnins.2014.00270

Bagatell, N. (2010). From cure to community: Transforming notions of autism. *Ethos, 38*(1), 33-55. https://doi.org/10.1111/j.1548-1352.2009.01080.x

Baldwin, S., Costley, D., & Warren, A. (2013). *We belong: The experiences, aspirations and needs of adults with Asperger's disorder and high functioning autism.* Aspect We Belong Research Report Issue. A. S. Australia.

Bargiela, S., Steward, R., & Mandy, W. (2016). The experiences of late-diagnosed women with Autism Spectrum Conditions: An investigation of the female autism phenotype. *Journal of Autism and Developmental Disorders, 46*(10), 3281-3294. https://doi.org/10.1007/s10803-016-2872-8

Baron-Cohen, S. (1997). *Mindblindness. An essay on autism and theory of mind.* The MIT Press.

Baron-Cohen, S. (2008). Theories of the autistic mind. *Psychologist, 21*(2), 112-116.

Baron-Cohen, S. (2015). ASD vs. ASC: Is one small letter important? Grand Ballroom B (Grand America Hotel).

Baron-Cohen, S., Wheelwright, S., Hill, J., Raste, Y., & Plumb, I. (2001). The 'reading the mind in the eyes' test revised version: A study

References

with normal adults, and adults with Asperger Syndrome or High-Functioning Autism. *Journal of Child Psychology and Psychiatry, 42*(2), 241-251. https://doi.org/10.1111/1469-7610.00715

Benning, S. D., Kovac, M., Campbell, A., Miller, S., Hanna, E. K., Damiano, C. R., Sabatino-DiCriscio, A., Turner-Brown, L., Sasson, N. J., Aaron, R. V., Kinard, J., & Dichter, G. S. (2016). Late positive potential ERP responses to social and nonsocial stimuli in youth with autism spectrum disorder. *Journal of Autism and Developmental Disorders, 46*(9), 3068-3077. https://doi.org/10.1007/s10803-016-2845-y

Berenguer, C., Miranda, A., Colomer, C., Baixauli, I., & Roselló, B. (2018). Contribution of theory of mind, executive functioning, and pragmatics to socialisation behaviours of children with high-functioning autism. *Journal of Autism and Developmental Disorders, 48*(2), 430-441. https://doi.org/10.1007/s10803-017-3349-0

Bolling, K. L. (2015). *Asperger's syndrome/autism spectrum disorder and marital satisfaction: A quantitative study.* Antioch University New England, Keene, New Hampshire.

Booth, R., Charlton, R., Hughes, C., & Happé, F. (2003). Disentangling weak coherence and executive dysfunction: planning drawing in autism and attention–deficit/hyperactivity disorder. *Philosophical Transactions of the Royal Society of London. Series B: Biological Sciences, 358*(1430), 387-392. https://doi.org/10.1098/rstb.2002.1204

Bos, A. E., Pryor, J. B., Reeder, G. D., & Stutterheim, S. E. (2013). Stigma: Advances in theory and research. *Basic and Applied Social Psychology, 35*(1), 1-9.

Bostock-Ling, J. S. (2017). *Life satisfaction of neurotypical women in intimate relationship with a partner who has Asperger's Syndrome: An exploratory study.* University of Sydney.

Bostock-Ling, J. S., Cumming, S. R., & Bundy, A. (2012). Life satisfaction of neurotypical women in intimate relationship with an Asperger's Syndrome partner: A systematic review of the literature. *Journal of Relationships Research, 3*(201212), 95-105. https://doi.org/10.1007/s10803-008-0541-2

Braden, B. B., Smith, C. J., Thompson, A., Glaspy, T. K., Wood, E., Vatsa, D., Abbott, A. E., McGee, S. C., & Baxter, L. C. (2017). Executive function and functional and structural brain differences in middle-age adults with autism spectrum disorder. *Autism Research, 10*(12), 1945-1959. https://doi.org/10.1002/aur.1842

Have We Gone Nuts?

Brady, D. I., Saklofske, D. H., Schwean, V. L., Montgomery, J. M., Thorne, K. J., & McCrimmon, A. W. (2017). Executive functions in young adults with autism spectrum disorder. *Focus on Autism and Other Developmental Disabilities, 32*(1), 31-43. https://doi.org/doi:10.1177/1088357615609306

Brewer, N., Young, R. L., & Barnett, E. (2017). Measuring Theory of Mind in adults with Autism Spectrum Disorder. *Journal of Autism and Developmental Disorders, 47*(7), 1927-1941. https://doi.org/10.1007/s10803-017-3080-x

Burnette, C., Mundy, P., Meyer, J., Sutton, S., Vaughan, A., & Charak, D. (2005). Weak central coherence and its relations to theory of mind and anxiety in autism. *Journal Autism Developmental Disorder, 35*(1), 63 -73.

Burrows, C. A., Usher, L. V., Mundy, P. C., & Henderson, H. A. (2017). The salience of the self: Self-referential processing and internalizing problems in children and adolescents with autism spectrum disorder. *Autism Research, 10*(5), 949-960. https://doi.org/10.1002/aur.1727

Cage, E., & Troxell-Whitman, Z. (2020). Understanding the relationships between autistic identity, disclosure, and camouflaging. *Autism Adulthood, 2*(4), 334-338. https://doi.org/10.1089/aut.2020.0016

Carpenter, B., Happé, F., & Egerton, J. (2019). *Girls and autism: Educational, family and personal perspectives.* Routledge.

Caruana, N., McArthur, G., Woolgar, A., & Brock, J. (2017). Simulating social interactions for the experimental investigation of joint attention. *Neuroscience & Biobehavioral Reviews, 74*(Part A), 115-125. https://doi.org/https://doi.org/10.1016/j.neubiorev.2016.12.022

Casanova, E. L., & Casanova, M. F. (2019). *Defining autism: a guide to brain, biology, and behavior.* Jessica Kingsley Publishers.

Casanova, M. (2019). Autism: Miswiring and misfiring in the cerebral cortex. https://www.ncsautism.org/blog/2019/2/21/autism-mis-wiring-and-mis-firing-in-the-cerebral-cortex

Catani, M., Dell'Acqua, F., Budisavljevic, S., Howells, H., Thiebaut de Schotten, M., Froudist-Walsh, S. n., D'Anna, L., Thompson, A., Sandrone, S., Bullmore, E. T., Suckling, J., Baron-Cohen, S., Lombardo, M. V., Wheelwright, S. J., Chakrabarti, B., Lai, M.-C., Ruigrok, A. N. V., Leemans, A., Ecker, C., . . . Murphy, D. G. M. (2016). Frontal networks in adults with autism spectrum disorder. *Brain: a journal of neurology, 139*(2), 616-630. https://doi.org/10.1093/brain/awv351

References

Ciaunica, A. (2019). The 'meeting of bodies': Empathy and basic forms of shared experiences. *Topoi: An International Review of Philosophy, 38*(1), 185-195. https://doi.org/10.1007/s11245-017-9500-x

Clutterbuck, R. A., Callan, M. J., Taylor, E. C., Livingston, L. A., & Shah, P. (2021). Development and validation of the four-item mentalising index. *Psychological Assessment, 33*(7), 629-636. https://doi.org/10.1037/pas0001004

Community Care Magazine. (2002). Living with Asperger's. *Community Care Magazine* (11), 38-39. http://www.communitycare.co.uk/2002/07/10/living-with-aspergers/

Cooke, A. N., Bazzini, D. G., Curtin, L. A., & Emery, L. J. (2018). Empathic understanding: Benefits of perspective-taking and facial mimicry instructions are mediated by self-other overlap. *Motivation and Emotion, 42*(3), 446-457. https://doi.org/10.1007/s11031-018-9671-9

Cooper, K., Smith, L. G. E., & Russell, A. (2017). Social identity, self-esteem, and mental health in autism. *European Journal of Social Psychology, 47*(7), 844-854. https://doi.org/10.1002/ejsp.2297

Coutelle, R., Goltzene, M.-A., Bizet, E., Schoenberger, M., Berna, F., & Danion, J.-M. (2020). Self-concept clarity and autobiographical memory functions in adults with Autism Spectrum Disorder without intellectual deficiency. *Journal of Autism and Developmental Disorders, 50*(11), 3874-3882.

Deisinger, J. A. (2011). Chapter 10: History of autism spectrum disorders. In A. Rotatori (Ed.), *History of Special Education* (Vol. 21, pp. 237-267): Emerald Group Publishing Limited.

den Houting, J. (2019). Neurodiversity: An insider's perspective. *Autism, 23*(2), 271-273. https://doi.org/10.1177/1362361318820762

Derlega, V. J. (2013). *Communication, intimacy, and close relationships.* Elsevier.

Dodd, S. (2005). *Understanding autism.* Elsevier Australia.

Doidge, N. (2007). *The brain that changes itself: Stories of personal triumph from the frontiers of brain science.* Penguin Group

Donovan, A. P., & Basson, M. A. (2017). The neuroanatomy of autism–a developmental perspective. *Journal of anatomy, 230*(1), 4-15.

Dritschel, B., Wisely, M., Goddard, L., Robinson, S., & Howlin, P. (2010). Judgements of self-understanding in adolescents with Asperger syndrome. *Autism, 14*(5), 509-518. https://doi.org/10.1177/1362361310368407

Dunn, D. S., & Andrews, E. E. (2015). Person-first and identity-first language: Developing psychologists' cultural competence using disability language. *The American Psychologist, 70*(3), 255-264.

Edwards, C., Love, A. M. A., Jones, S. C., Cai, R. Y., Nguyen, B. T. H., & Gibbs, V. (2023). 'Most people have no idea what autism is': Unpacking autism disclosure using social media analysis. *Autism.* https://doi.org/10.1177/13623613231192133

Edwards, D. (2008). *Providing practical support for people with autism spectrum disorder: Supported living in the community.* Jessica Kingsley Publishers.

Eid, P., & Boucher, S. (2012). Alexithymia and dyadic adjustment in intimate relationships: Analyses using the actor partner interdependence model. *Journal of Social and Clinical Psychology, 31*(10), 1095-1111. https://doi.org/101521jscp201231101095

Elder, J., & Thomas, M. (2006). *Different like me: My book of autism heroes.* Jessica Kingsley. http://catdir.loc.gov/catdir/toc/ecip0512/2005014169.html

Feng, X., Sun, B., Chen, C., Li, W., Wang, Y., Zhang, W., Xiao, W., & Shao, Y. (2020). Self–other overlap and interpersonal neural synchronization serially mediate the effect of behavioral synchronization on prosociality. *Social Cognitive and Affective Neuroscience, 15*(2), 203-214.

Finke, E. H. (2023). The kind of friend I think I am: Perceptions of autistic and non-autistic young adults. *Journal of Autism and Developmental Disorders, 53*(8), 3047-3064. https://doi.org/10.1007/s10803-022-05573-4

Fitzgerald, M. (2020). *Empathy Study.* IntechOpen. https://doi.org/10.5772/intechopen.76278

Fletcher-Watson, S., Leekam, S. R., & Findlay, J. M. (2013). Social interest in high-functioning adults with Autism Spectrum Disorders. *Focus on Autism and Other Developmental Disabilities, 28*(4), 222-229. https://doi.org/10.1177/1088357613480829

Galinsky, A. D., Ku, G., & Wang, C. S. (2005). Perspective-taking and self-other overlap: Fostering social bonds and facilitating social coordination. *Group Processes & Intergroup Relations, 8*(2), 109-124.

Garon, N., Zwaigenbaum, L., Bryson, S. E., Smith, I. M., Brian, J., Roncadin, C., Vaillancourt, T., Armstrong, V. L., Sacrey, L.-A. R., & Roberts, W. (2022). Precursors of self-regulation in infants at elevated likelihood for autism spectrum disorder. *Developmental Science, 25*(5). https://doi.org/10.1111/desc.13247

References

Gottman, J., & Gottman, J. (2017). The natural principles of love. *Journal of Family Theory & Review, 9*(1), 7-26. https://doi.org/10.1111/jftr.12182

Graham, S. M., & Clark, M. S. (2006). Self-esteem and organization of valenced information about others: The 'Jekyll and Hyde'-ing of relationship Partners. *Journal of Personality and Social Psychology, 90*(4), 652-665.

Granader, Y., Wallace, G. L., Hardy, K. K., Yerys, B. E., Lawson, R. A., Rosenthal, M., Wills, M. C., Dixon, E., Pandey, J., Penna, R., Schultz, R. T., & Kenworthy, L. (2014). Characterizing the factor structure of parent reported Executive Function in autism spectrum disorders: The impact of cognitive inflexibility. *Journal of Autism and Developmental Disorders, 44*(12), 3056-3062. https://doi.org/10.1007/s10803-014-2169-8

Gurash, N. (2023). So...What is Cassandra Syndrome, Anyway? https://spectrumconnecttherapy.com/so-what-is-cassandra-syndrome-anyway/

Han, E., Scior, K., Heath, E., Umagami, K., & Crane, L. (2023). Development of stigma-related support for autistic adults: Insights from the autism community. *Autism, 27*(6), 1676-1689. https://doi.org/10.1177/13623613221143590

Happé, F., Booth, R., Charlton, R., & Hughes, C. (2006). Executive function deficits in autism spectrum disorders and attention-deficit/hyperactivity disorder: Examining profiles across domains and ages. *Brain and Cognition, 61*(1), 25-39. https://doi.org/10.1016/j.bandc.2006.03.004

Happé, F., & Frith, U. (2006). The weak coherence account: Detail-focused cognitive style in Autism Spectrum Disorders. *Journal of Autism and Developmental Disorders, 36*(1), 5-25. https://doi.org/10.1007/s10803-005-0039-0

Haslam, C., Cruwys, T., Haslam, S. A., & Jetten, J. (2015). Social connectedness and health. *Encyclopedia of geropsychology, 46*(1), 1-10.

Hassan, A., & Barber, S. J. (2021). The effects of repetition frequency on the illusory truth effect. *Cognitive research: principles and implications, 6*(1), 1-12.

Heasman, B., & Gillespie, A. (2017). Perspective-taking is two-sided: Misunderstandings between people with Asperger's syndrome and their family members. *Autism, 22*(6), 740-750. https://doi.org/10.1177/1362361317708287

Howlin, P., & Magiati, I. (2017). Autism spectrum disorder: outcomes in adulthood. *Current Opinion in Psychiatry, 30*(2), 69-76. https://doi.org/org/10.1097/YCO.0000000000000308

Huang, A. X., Hughes, T. L., Sutton, L. R., Lawrence, M., Chen, X., Ji, Z., & Zeleke, W. (2017). Understanding the self in individuals with Autism Spectrum Disorders (ASD): A review of literature. *Frontiers in psychology, 8*, 1422. https://doi.org/10.3389/fpsyg.2017.01422

Huggins, C. F., Donnan, G., Cameron, I. M., & Williams, J. H. (2021). Emotional self-awareness in autism: A meta-analysis of group differences and developmental effects. *Autism, 25*(2), 307-321. https://doi.org/10.1177/1362361320964306

Hughes, C., & Leekam, S. (2004). What are the Links Between Theory of Mind and Social Relations? Review, Reflections and New Directions for Studies of Typical and Atypical Development [Journal]. *Social Development, 13*(4), 590-619. https://doi.org/10.1111/j.1467-9507.2004.00285.x

Hull, L., Petrides, K. V., Allison, C., Smith, P., Baron-Cohen, S., Lai, M.-C., & Mandy, W. (2017). 'Putting on my best normal': Social camouflaging in adults with autism spectrum conditions. *Journal of Autism and Developmental Disorders, 47*(8), 2519-2534.

Hwang, Y. I., Arnold, S., Srasuebkul, P., & Trollor, J. (2020). Understanding anxiety in adults on the autism spectrum: An investigation of its relationship with intolerance of uncertainty, sensory sensitivities and repetitive behaviours. *Autism, 24*(2), 411-422. https://doi.org/10.1177/1362361319868907

Ibrahim, K., Kalvin, C., Marsh, C. L., Anzano, A., Gorynova, L., Cimino, K., & Sukhodolsky, D. G. (2019). Anger rumination is associated with restricted and repetitive behaviors in children with autism spectrum disorder. *Journal of Autism and Developmental Disorders, 49*(9), 3656-3668. https://doi.org/10.1007/s10803-019-04085-y

James, I. (2005). *Asperger's Syndrome and high achievement: Some very remarkable people.* Jessica Kingsley Publishers. https://ebookcentral.proquest.com/lib/ECU/detail.action?docID=290867

Johnston, K., Murray, K., Spain, D., Walker, I., & Russell, A. (2019). Executive Function: Cognition and behaviour in adults with autism spectrum disorders (ASD). *Journal of Autism and Developmental Disorders, 49*(10), 4181-4192. https://doi.org/10.1007/s10803-019-04133-7

Joseph, R. M., & Tager-Flusberg, H. (2004). The relationship of theory of mind and executive functions to symptom type and severity in children with autism. *Development and Psychopatholy, 16*(1), 137-155. https://doi.org/10.1017/s095457940404444x

Jurado, M. B., & Rosselli, M. (2007). The elusive nature of executive functions: A review of our current understanding. *Neuropsychology Review, 17,* 213-233. https://doi.org/10.1007/s11065-007-9040-z

Kapp, S. K., Gillespie-Lynch, K., Sherman, L. E., & Hutman, T. (2013). Deficit, difference, or both? Autism and neurodiversity. *Developmental Psychology, 49*(1), 59-71.

Karwowski, M., & Kaufman, J. C. (2017). *The creative self: Effect of beliefs, self-efficacy, mindset, and identity.* Elsevier Science. https://www.sciencedirect.com/science/book/9780128097908

Keenan, E. G., Gotham, K., & Lerner, M. D. (2018). Hooked on a feeling: Repetitive cognition and internalizing symptomatology in relation to autism spectrum symptomatology. *Autism: the international journal of research and practice, 22*(7), 814-824. https://doi.org/10.1177/1362361317709603

Keysar, B., Converse, B. A., Wang, J., & Epley, N. (2008). Reciprocity is not give and take: Asymmetric reciprocity to positive and negative acts. *Psychological Science, 19*(12), 1280-1286. https://doi.org/10.1111/j.1467-9280.2008.02223.x

Kimura, Y., Fujioka, T., Jung, M., Fujisawa, T. X., Tomoda, A., & Kosaka, H. (2020). An investigation of the effect of social reciprocity, social anxiety, and letter fluency on communicative behaviors in adults with autism spectrum disorder. *Psychiatry Research 294,* 113503. https://doi.org/10.1016/j.psychres.2020.113503

Kinnear, S. H., Link, B. G., Ballan, M. S., & Fischbach, R. L. (2016). Understanding the experience of stigma for parents of children with autism spectrum disorder and the role stigma plays in families' lives. *Journal of Autism and Developmental Disorders, 46*(3), 942-953. https://doi.org/10.1007/s10803-015-2637-9

Koffer Miller, K. H., Mathew, M., Nonnemacher, S. L., & Shea, L. L. (2018). Program experiences of adults with autism, their families, and providers: Findings from a focus group study. *Autism, 22*(3), 345-356. https://doi.org/10.1177/1362361316679000

Koldewyn, K., Jiang, Y. V., Weigelt, S., & Kanwisher, N. (2013). Global/local processing in autism: Not a disability, but a disinclination. *Journal of Autism and Developmental Disorders, 43*(10), 2329-2340. https://doi.org/10.1007/s10803-013-1777-z

Kosger, F., Sevil, S., Subasi, Z., & Kaptanoglu, C. (2015). Asperger's Syndrome in adulthood: A case report/Eriskin Asperger Sendromu: Olgu sunumu. *Dusunen Adam, 28*(4), 382-386. https://doi.org/10.5350/DAJPN2015280408

Kushki, A., Cardy, R. E., Panahandeh, S., Malihi, M., Hammill, C., Brian, J., Iaboni, A., Taylor, M. J., Schachar, R., Crosbie, J., Arnold, P., Kelley, E., Ayub, M., Nicolson, R., Georgiades, S., Lerch, J. P., & Anagnostou, E. (2021). Cross-diagnosis structural correlates of autistic-like social communication differences. *Cerebral Cortex, 31*(11), 5067-5076. https://doi.org/10.1093/cercor/bhab142

Lai, M.-C., & Baron-Cohen, S. (2015). Identifying the lost generation of adults with autism spectrum conditions. *The lancet. Psychiatry, 2*(11), 1013-1027. https://doi.org/org/10.1016/S2215-0366(15)00277-1

Laurenceau, J.-P., Pietromonaco, P. R., & Barrett, L. F. (1998). Intimacy as an interpersonal process: the importance of self-disclosure, partner disclosure, and perceived partner responsiveness in interpersonal exchanges. *Journal of Personality and Social Psychology, 74*(5), 1238-1251.

Leadbitter, K., Buckle, K. L., Ellis, C., & Dekker, M. (2021). Autistic self-advocacy and the neurodiversity movement: Implications for autism early intervention research and practice. *Frontiers in psychology, 12.* https://doi.org/10.3389/fpsyg.2021.635690

Lehnhardt, F.-G., Gawronski, A., Pfeiffer, K., Kockler, H., Schilbach, L., & Vogeley, K. (2013). The investigation and differential diagnosis of Asperger Syndrome in adults. *Deutsches Ärzteblatt International, 110*(45), 755-763. https://doi.org/10.3238/arztebl.2013.0755

León, F. (2019). Autism, social connectedness, and minimal social acts. *Adaptive Behavior, 27*(1), 75-89. https://doi.org/10.1177/1059712318818813

Lever, A. G., & Geurts, H. M. (2016). Age-related differences in cognition across the adult lifespan in autism spectrum disorder. *Autism Research, 9*(6), 666-676. https://doi.org/10.1002/aur.1545

Lewis, L. F., & Stevens, K. (2023). The lived experience of meltdowns for autistic adults. *Autism.* https://doi.org/10.1177/13623613221145783

Lind, S. E., & Bowler, D. M. (2009). Delayed self-recognition in children with autism spectrum disorder. *Journal of Autism and Developmental Disorders, 39*(4), 643-650. https://doi.org/10.1007/s10803-008-0670-7

Lipinski, S., Blanke, E. S., Suenkel, U., & Dziobek, I. (2019). Outpatient Psychotherapy for Adults with High-Functioning Autism Spectrum Condition: Utilization, Treatment Satisfaction, and Preferred Modifications.

References

Journal of Autism and Developmental Disorders, 49(3), 1154-1168. https://doi. org/10.1007/s10803-018-3797-1

Lipinski, S., Boegl, K., Blanke, E. S., Suenkel, U., & Dziobek, I. (2021). A blind spot in mental healthcare? Psychotherapists lack education and expertise for the support of adults on the autism spectrum. *Autism, 26*(6), 1509-1521. https://doi.org/10.1177/13623613211057973

Liu, M. Y. (2014). *Psychological self-other overlap: Implications for prosocial behavior in close relationships*

Lockwood, P. L., Ang, Y.-S., Husain, M., & Crockett, M. J. (2017). Individual differences in empathy are associated with apathy-motivation. *Scientific Reports, 7*(1).

Lombardo, M. V., & Baron-Cohen, S. (2011). The role of the self in mindblindness in autism. *Consciousness and Cognition, 20*(1), 130-140. https://doi.org/10.1016/j.concog.2010.09.006

Lorant, J. B. (2011). *Impact on emotional connectivity in couples in which one partner has Asperger's Syndrome* Alliant International University]. WorldCat.org. https://www.proquest.com/dissertations-theses/ impact-on-emotional-connectivity-couples-which/docview/880566433/ se-2

Loth, E., Gómez, J. C., & Happé, F. (2010). When seeing depends on knowing: Adults with Autism Spectrum Conditions show diminished top-down processes in the visual perception of degraded faces but not degraded objects. *Neuropsychologia, 48*(5), 1227-1236. https://doi.org/ http://dx.doi.org/10.1016/j.neuropsychologia.2009.12.023

Lovett, J. P. (2005). *Solutions for adults with Asperger Syndrome. Maximizing the benefits, minimizing the drawbacks to achieve success.* Fair Winds Press.

Lyons, V., & Fitzgerald, M. (2013). Atypical sense of self in autism spectrum disorders: A neuro-cognitive perspective. In *Recent Advances in Autism Spectrum Disorders-Volume I*. IntechOpen.

Mandy, W. (2019). Social camouflaging in autism: Is it time to lose the mask? *Autism, 23*(8), 1879-1881. https://doi.org/10.1177/1362361319878559

Markus, H., & Wurf, E. (1987). The dynamic self-concept: A social psychological perspective. *Annual Review of Psychology, 38*(1), 299-337.

Mashek, D. J., & Aron, A. (2004). *Handbook of closeness and intimacy.* Lawrence Erlbaum Associates. https://public.ebookcentral.proquest. com/choice/publicfullrecord.aspx?p=335513

McKenzie, K., Russell, A., Golm, D., & Fairchild, G. (2021). Empathic accuracy and cognitive and affective empathy in young adults with and without autism spectrum disorder. *Journal of Autism and Developmental Disorders, 52*(5), 2004-2018. https://doi.org/10.1007/s10803-021-05093-7

Mendes, E. (2015). *Marriage and lasting relationships with Asperger's Syndrome (Autism Spectrum Disorder): Successful strategies for couples or counselors.* Jessica Kingsley Publishers.

Millar-Powell, N., & Warburton, W. A. (2020). Caregiver burden and relationship satisfaction in ASD-NT relationships. *Journal of Relationships Research, 11*(e15), 1-8. https://doi.org/10.1017/jrr.2020.11

Mitran, C. L. (2022). A new framework for examining impact of neurodiversity in couples in intimate relationships. *The Family Journal, 30*(3), 437-443. https://doi.org/10.1177/10664807211063194

Montebarocci, O., Surcinelli, P., Rossi, N., & Baldaro, B. (2011). Alexithymia, verbal ability and emotion recognition. *Psychiatric Quarterly, 82*(3), 245-252. https://doi.org/http://dx.doi.org/10.1007/s11126-010-9166-7

Nadig, A., Lee, I., Singh, L., Bosshart, K., & Ozonoff, S. (2010). How does the topic of conversation affect verbal exchange and eye gaze? A comparison between typical development and high-functioning autism. *Neuropsychologia, 48*(9), 2730-2739. https://doi.org/10.1016/j.neuropsychologia.2010.05.020

Nguyen, W., Ownsworth, T., Nicol, C., & Zimmerman, D. (2020). How I see and feel about myself: domain-specific self-concept and self-esteem in autistic adults. *Frontiers in Psychology, 11*, 913.

Nicolaidis, C. (2019). Autism in adulthood: The new home for our emerging field. Autism Adulthood, (Vol. 1, pp. 1-3).

Ozsivadjian, A., Hollocks, M. J., Magiati, I., Happé, F., Baird, G., & Absoud, M. (2021). Is cognitive inflexibility a missing link? The role of cognitive inflexibility, alexithymia and intolerance of uncertainty in externalising and internalising behaviours in young people with autism spectrum disorder. *Journal of Child Psychology and Psychiatry, 62*(6), 715-724. https://doi.org/10.1111/jcpp.13295

Parise, M., Pagani, A. F., Donato, S., & Sedikides, C. (2019). Self-concept clarity and relationship satisfaction at the dyadic level. *Personal Relationships, 26*(1), 54-72. https://doi.org/10.1111/pere.12265

Patel, S., Day, T. N., Jones, N., & Mazefsky, C. A. (2017). Association between anger rumination and autism symptom severity, depression

References

symptoms, aggression, and general dysregulation in adolescents with autism spectrum disorder. *Autism, 21*(2), 181-189. https://doi.org/10.1177/1362361316633566

Pellicano, E., Dinsmore, A., & Charman, T. (2014). What should autism research focus upon? Community views and priorities from the United Kingdom. *Autism, 18*(7), 756-770. https://doi.org/10.1177/1362361314529627

Pelzl, M. A., Travers-Podmaniczky, G., Brück, C., Jacob, H., Hoffmann, J., Martinelli, A., Hölz, L., Wabersich-Flad, D., & Wildgruber, D. (2022). Reduced impact of nonverbal cues during integration of verbal and nonverbal emotional information in adults with high-functioning autism. *Frontiers in Psychiatry, 13*, 1069028. https://doi.org/10.3389/fpsyt.2022.1069028

Petrolini, V., Jorba, M., & Vicente, A. (2023). What does it take to be rigid? Reflections on the notion of rigidity in autism. *Frontiers in Psychiatry, 14*, 1072362.

Powell, P. S., Klinger, L. G., & Klinger, M. R. (2017). Patterns of age-related cognitive differences in adults with autism spectrum disorder. *Journal of Autism and Developmental Disorders, 47*(10), 3204-3219. https://doi.org/10.1007/s10803-017-3238-6

Premack, D., & Woodruff, G. (1978). Does the chimpanzee have a theory of mind. *The Behavioural and Brain Sciences, 4*, 515-525.

Pugliese, C. E., Anthony, L. G., Strang, J. F., Dudley, K., Wallace, G. L., Naiman, D. Q., & Kenworthy, L. (2016). Longitudinal examination of adaptive behavior in autism spectrum disorders: influence of Executive Function. *Journal of Autism and Developmental Disorders, 46*(2), 467-477. https://doi.org/10.1007/s10803-015-2584-5

Pugliese, C. E., Fritz, M. S., & White, S. W. (2014). The role of anger rumination and autism spectrum disorder–linked perseveration in the experience of aggression in the general population. *Autism, 00*(0), 1-9. https://doi.org/10.1177/1362361314548731

Quintard, V., Jouffe, S., Hommel, B., & Bouquet, C. A. (2020). Embodied self-other overlap in romantic love: a review and integrative perspective. *Psychological research*, 1-16.

Redelmeier, D. A., & Ng, K. (2020). Approach to making the availability heuristic less available. *BMJ Quality & Safety, 29*(7), 528-530. https://doi.org/10.1136/bmjqs-2020-010831

Rench, C. (2014). *When eros meets autos: Marriage to someone with autism spectrum disorder* Doctoral dissertation, Capella University.

ProQuest Dissertations Publishing. https://www.proquest.com/dissertations-theses/when-i-eros-meets-autos-marriage-someone-with/docview/1656449694/se-2

Robic, S., Sonié, S., Fonlupt, P., Henaff, M.-A., Touil, N., Coricelli, G., Mattout, J., & Schmitz, C. (2015). Decision-making in a changing world: A study in Autism Spectrum Disorders. *Journal of Autism and Developmental Disorders, 45*(6), 1603-1613. https://doi.org/10.1007/s10803-014-2311-7

Rodgers, J., Herrema, R., Honey, E., & Freeston, M. (2018). Towards a treatment for intolerance of uncertainty for autistic adults: A single case experimental design study. *Journal of Autism and Developmental Disorders, 48*, 2832-2845.

Rodman, K. E. (2003). *Asperger's Syndome and adults … Is anyone listening?* Jessica Kingsley Publishers.

Rueda, P., Fernández-Berrocal, P., & Baron-Cohen, S. (2015). Dissociation between cognitive and affective empathy in youth with Asperger Syndrome. *European Journal of Developmental Psychology, 12*(1), 85-98.

Russell, G., & Lightman, S. (2019). The human stress response. *Nature reviews. Endocrinology, 15*(9), 525-534. https://doi.org/10.1038/s41574-019-0228-0

Sachdeva, N., & Jones, G. (2018). Diagnosis of autism in adulthood: What can we learn? *Good Autism Practice, 19*(2), 63-74.

Sakellariadis, A. (2011). A wider sense of normal? Seeking to understand Pierre Rivière through the lens of autism. *Emotion, Space and Society, 00*(0), 1-10. https://doi.org/10.1016/j.emospa.2012.03.003

Sasson, N. J., & Morrison, K. E. (2019). First impressions of adults with autism improve with diagnostic disclosure and increased autism knowledge of peers. *Autism: The International Journal of Research and Practice, 23*(1), 50-59.

Sato, W., Kochiyama, T., Uono, S., Yoshimura, S., Kubota, Y., Sawada, R., Sakihama, M., & Toichi, M. (2017). Reduced gray matter volume in the social brain network in adults with Autism Spectrum Disorder. *Frontiers in Human Neuroscience, 11*(395), 1-12. https://doi.org/10.3389/fnhum.2017.00395

Schaller, U. M., & Rauh, R. (2017). What difference does it make? Implicit, explicit and complex social cognition in Autism Spectrum Disorders. *Journal of Autism and Developmental Disorders, 47*(4), 961-979. https://doi.org/10.1007/s10803-016-3008-x

References

Shakes, P., & Cashin, A. (2019). Identifying language for people on the autism spectrum: A scoping review. *Issues in Mental Health Nursing*, *40*(4), 317-325. https://doi.org/10.1080/01612840.2018.1522400

Showers, C. J., & Zeigler-Hill, V. (2007). Compartmentalization and integration: The evaluative organization of contextualized selves. *Journal of Personality*, *75*(6), 1181-1204. https://doi.org/10.1111/j.1467-6494.2007.00472.x

Simone, R. (2010). *Aspergirls: Empowering females with Asperger Syndrome.* Jessica Kingsley Publishers.

Simons, H. F., & Thompson, J. R. (2009). Affective deprivation disorder: Does it constitute a relational disorder. *Affective deprivation disorder.*

Smith, A. (2009). The empathy imbalance hypothesis of autism: A theoretical approach to cognitive and emotional empathy in autistic development. *The Psychological Record*, *59*(3), 489-510. https://doi.org/10.1007/BF03395675

Smith, O., & Jones, S. C. (2020). 'Coming out' with autism: Identity in people with an Asperger's diagnosis after DSM-5. *Journal of Autism and Developmental Disorders*, *50*(2), 592-602. https://doi.org/10.1007/s10803-019-04294-5

Smith, R., Netto, J., Gribble, N. C., & Falkmer, M. (2020). 'At the end of the day, it's love': An exploration of relationships in neurodiverse couples. *Journal of Autism and Developmental Disorders*, *51*, 3311-3321. https://doi.org/10.1007/s10803-020-04790-z

Song, Y., Nie, T., Shi, W., Zhao, X., & Yang, Y. (2019). Empathy impairment in individuals with autism spectrum conditions from a multidimensional perspective: A meta-analysis. *10.*

Stagg, S. D., & Belcher, H. (2019). Living with autism without knowing: receiving a diagnosis in later life. *Health Psychology and Behavioral Medicine*, *7*(1), 348-361. https://doi.org/10.1080/21642850.2019.1684920

Stark, E., & Hester, M. (2018). Coercive control: Update and review. *Violence Against Women*, *25*(1), 81-104. https://doi.org/10.1177/1077801218816191

Stroebe, M., Schut, H., & Boerner, K. (2017). Cautioning health-care professionals: Bereaved persons are misguided through the stages of grief. *OMEGA - Journal of Death and Dying*, *74*(4), 455-473. https://doi.org/10.1177/0030222817691870

Strunz, R. M. (2018). Common factors of a transtheoretical model of Autism Spectrum Disorder-informed psychotherapy. *Canadian Journal of Counselling and Psychotherapy*, *52*(3).

Tantam, D. (2012). *Autism Spectrum Disorders through the life span.* Jessica Kingsley Publishers.

Tierney, S., Burns, J., & Kilbey, E. (2016). Looking behind the mask: Social coping strategies of girls on the autistic spectrum. *Research in Autism Spectrum Disorders, 23*, 73-83.

Tili, T. R., & Barker, G. G. (2015). Communication in intercultural marriages: Managing cultural differences and conflicts. *Southern Communication Journal, 80*(3), 189-210. https://doi.org/10.1080/1041794X.2015.1023826

Townsend, A. N., Guzick, A. G., Hertz, A. G., Kerns, C. M., Goodman, W. K., Berry, L. N., Kendall, P. C., Wood, J. J., & Storch, E. A. (2022). Anger Outbursts in Youth with ASD and Anxiety: Phenomenology and Relationship with Family Accommodation. *Child Psychiatry and Human Development.* https://doi.org/10.1007/s10578-022-01489-3

Tsai, L. Y. (2013). Asperger's disorder will be back. *Journal of Autism and Developmental Disorders, 43*(12), 2914-2942. https://doi.org/http://dx.doi.org/10.1007/s10803-013-1839-2

Uddin, L. Q. (2011). The self in autism: An emerging view from neuroimaging. *Neurocase, 17*(3), 201-208. https://doi.org/10.1080/13554794.2010.509320

Vandervoort, D., & Rokach, A. (2004). Abusive relationships: Is a new category for traumatization needed? *Current Psychology, 23*(1), 68-76.

Vermeulen, P. (2012). *Autism as context blindness.* AAPC Publishing.

Vermeulen, P. (2015). Context blindness in autism spectrum disorder not using the forest to see the trees as trees. *Focus on Autism and Other Developmental Disabilities, 30*(3), 182-192. https://doi.org/10.1177/1088357614528799

Wainer, A. L., Hepburn, S., & Griffith, E. M. (2017). Remembering parents in parent-mediated early intervention: An approach to examining impact on parents and families. *Autism, 21*(1), 5-17. https://doi.org/doi:10.1177/1362361315622411

Warfield, M. E., Crossman, M. K., Delahaye, J., Der Weerd, E., & Kuhlthau, K. A. (2015). Physician perspectives on providing primary medical care to adults with autism spectrum disorders (ASD). *Journal of Autism and Developmental Disorders, 45*(7), 2209-2217. https://doi.org/10.1007/s10803-015-2386-9

Waugh, C. E., & Fredrickson, B. L. (2006). Nice to know you: Positive emotions, self–other overlap, and complex understanding in the

References

formation of a new relationship. *The Journal of Positive Psychology, 1*(2), 93-106.

Webster, G. D., Brunell, A. B., & Pilkington, C. J. (2009). Individual differences in men's and women's warmth and disclosure differentially moderate couples' reciprocity in conversational disclosure. *Personality and Individual Differences, 46*(3), 292-297. https://doi.org/https://doi.org/10.1016/j.paid.2008.10.014

Weinstein, N., Rodriguez, L. M., Knee, C. R., & Kumashiro, M. (2016). Self-determined self-other overlap: Interacting effects on partners' perceptions of support and well-being in close relationships. *Journal of Research in Personality, 65*, 130-139. https://doi.org/10.1016/j.jrp.2016.10.011

Westby, C. (2017). Autism as a problem of context blindness. *Word of Mouth, 28*(5), 8-12. https://doi.org/10.1177/1048395017705385b

White, S. W., Scarpa, A., Conner, C. M., Maddox, B. B., & Bonete, S. (2015). Evaluating change in social skills in high-functioning adults with autism spectrum disorder using a laboratory-based observational measure. *Focus on Autism and Other Developmental Disabilities, 30*(1), 3-12. https://doi.org/doi:10.1177/1088357614539836

Wilkinson, L. A. (2016, Thursday, June 30, 2016). Alexithymia, empathy, and autism. http://bestpracticeautism.blogspot.com.au/2012/02/alexithymia-empathy-and-autism.html

Williams, D. (2010). Theory of own mind in autism: Evidence of a specific deficit in self-awareness? *Autism, 14*(5), 474-494. https://doi.org/10.1177/1362361310366314

Williams, D. M., Nicholson, T., & Grainger, C. (2018). The self-reference effect on perception: Undiminished in adults with autism and no relation to autism traits. *Autism Research, 11*(2), 331-341. https://doi.org/10.1002/aur.1891

Williams, E. (2004). Who really needs a 'theory' of mind? *Theory & Psychology, 14*(5), 704-724. https://doi.org/10.1177/0959354304046180

Williams, Z. J., Everaert, J., & Gotham, K. O. (2021). Measuring depression in autistic adults: Psychometric validation of the Beck Depression Inventory-II. *Assessment, 28*(3), 858-876. https://doi.org/10.1177/1073191120952889

Woodman, A. C., Mailick, M. R., & Greenberg, J. S. (2016). Trajectories of internalizing and externalizing symptoms among adults with autism spectrum disorders. *Development and Psychopatholy, 28*(2), 565-581. https://doi.org/10.1017/s095457941500108x

Zeestraten, E. A., Gudbrandsen, M. C., Daly, E., de Schotten, M. T., Catani, M., Dell'Acqua, F., Lai, M. C., Ruigrok, A. N. V., Lombardo, M. V., Chakrabarti, B., Baron-Cohen, S., Ecker, C., Consortium, M. A., Anthony, J. B., Simon, B.-C., Patrick, F. B., Edward, T. B., Sarah, C., Marco, C., . . . Craig, M. C. (2017). Sex differences in frontal lobe connectivity in adults with autism spectrum conditions. *Translational Psychiatry, 7*(e1090), 1-8.

Zerbo, O., Massolo, M. L., Qian, Y., & Croen, L. A. (2015). A study of physician knowledge and experience with autism in adults in a large integrated healthcare system. *Journal of Autism and Developmental Disorders, 45*(12), 4002-4014. https://doi.org/10.1007/s10803-015-2579-2

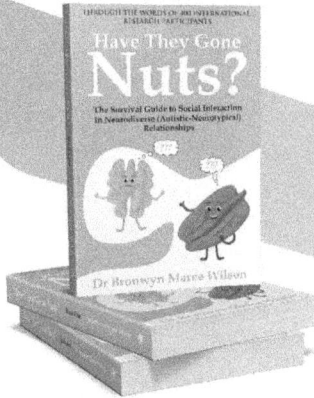

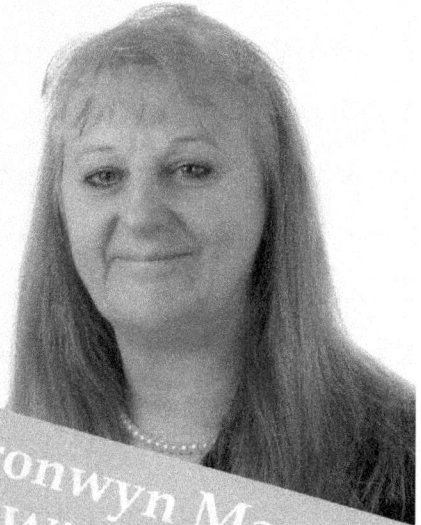

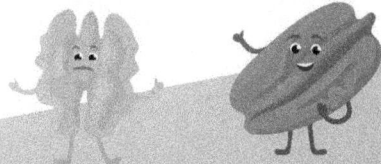

281

About the Author

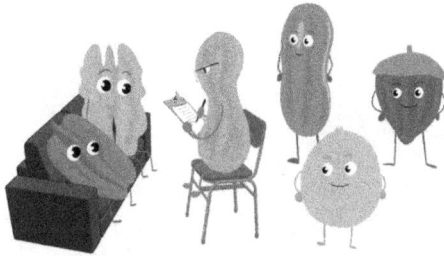

Bronwyn Wilson lives in a small beachside town in Western Australia, after moving from Queensland for her husband's work. Following a career in teaching she embarked on research, completing a PhD thesis at Edith Cowan University, Perth, Western Australia, researching the communication difficulties that can occur within the close relationships of adults with ASD Level 1 (Asperger's Syndrome). Bronwyn also holds a Master of Special Education, obtained from Griffith University, Brisbane, and a Bachelor of Education, obtained from James Cook University, Townsville.

She has published peer-reviewed papers and presented at the 5th Asia Pacific Autism Conference in 2017 held at the International Convention Centre in Sydney, and at the 5th World Autism Conference, Houston, Texas, USA in 2018. Today, Bronwyn works as an online sessional tutor at Edith Cowan University while also authoring books and journal articles. She enjoys swimming most days, sewing and decorating her home, along with watching the boats go past, listening to the waves and enjoying the ocean views from her verandah.

Growing The Knowing Learning Modules

12 Steps to Becoming a More Knowing You

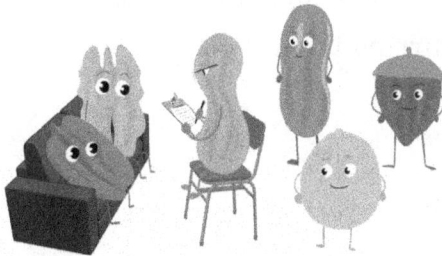

These learning modules are aligned to the book. Evidence suggests that ASC and NT adults have even greater differences compared to individuals from completely different cultures (Grigg, 2012; Rodman, 2003; Smith et al., 2020). When added together these differences collectively establish its own culture. The culture of the neurodiverse relationship, therefore, is like no other relationship. However, the more informed we are, the better prepared we are to make informed choices. For those who have a desire to know more, to dig deeper and to improve your understanding of the differences and difficulties specific to the neurodiverse relationship, these modules provide additional information on each topic covered in this book. Plus, a few extra bonus topics are also included.

285

Have We Gone Nuts?

The more we know the more we grow. To get started go to the Growing the Knowing Learning Modules tab on the website –bronwilson.com

MODULE ONE: Climbing The Awareness Ladder

- The Evolution of Understanding
- Generation Lost
- Debates, Doubts and Diagnosis
- The Pros and Cons of a Diagnosis
- Co-occurring Conditions
- Levels of Autism

MODULE TWO: Dancing With Difference

- The Differences in Brain Wiring
- A Dance of Different Brains
- A Reciprocity Side-Step
- Dancing Alone
- Movement Profiles
- Social Knowledge Gaps

MODULE THREE: A Mysterious Blindness

- The Innermost Recesses
- Thinking Absolutely
- Attention to Detail
- Captivated by Specialties
- Self/Other Understandings
- The Self-Other Overlap

MODULE FOUR: Associated Anomalies

- A Matter of Monologues
- The Perseverative Predicament
- A Depression Dilemma
- A Tendency Toward Helplessness
- The Non-Verbal Drawback
- Intolerances of Uncertainty

MODULE FIVE: A Toxic Tailspin

- Features of Adaptive Behaviour
- The Presence of Rage Attacks
- Matters of Meltdown
- Matters of Maltreatment
- Regulating by Rules
- Managing by Mandates

MODULE SIX: Needs Deprivation

- A Needs Divergence
- The Many Sides of Empathy
- A Question of Disinclination
- Incongruent Preferences
- Contrasting Perceptions
- Competing Partnerships

MODULE SEVEN: Heed Cassandra's Warning

- Cassandra's Controversy
- Cassandra's Clues
- A Need to Believe
- The Sorrow of Scepticism
- Loneliness and Isolation
- Considering Cassandras

MODULE EIGHT: Conspiracies Of Silence

- Struggling with Stigma
- Camouflaging and Concealing
- Disclosure Dilemmas
- Hidden Consequences
- Revelation's Rewards
- Reversing Discrimination

MODULE NINE: Clinical Complications

- The Research Gap
- The Knowledge and Intervention Gap
- Counter-Therapeutic Practices
- Reversing Clinician Reservations
- The Change Challenge
- Advancing Appropriate Assessments

Growing The Knowing Learning Modules

MODULE TEN: A Double-Edged Sword

- A Service Cliff
- Building Essential Services
- Building Essential Training
- Factors For Consideration
- Prerequisites for Targeted Support
- Towards Combined Support

MODULE ELEVEN: Seeking An Urgent Upgrade

- Surprising Similarities
- Divisions of Difference
- Promoting Education
- Advancing Awareness
- Participant Perspectives
- Designing Interventions

MODULE TWELVE: Steps Forward

- Healthy and Unhealthy Patterns
- Fundamentals of Change
- Educating Ourselves
- Educating Others
- In a Nutshell
- Final Thoughts

Acknowledgements

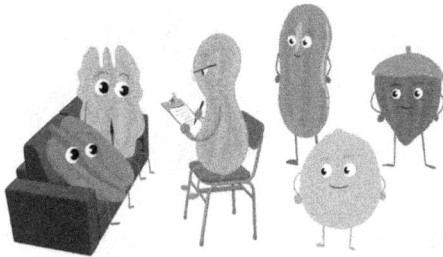

I express my sincere gratitude to each of my supervisors who supported me in my studies – Dr Wendi Beamish and Dr Steve Hay in the first, and Dr Susan Main, Dr John O'Rourke and Dr Deslea Konza in the second. Their professional and personal commitment, and their input and feedback, assisted in the realisation of research that I am honoured to have accomplished. Their valuable support has contributed to raising awareness of the unseen struggles of the population of people whose life challenges were explored in these studies.

A special mention goes to Professor Tony Attwood; a wise and knowledgeable supporter of my research journey, who, over quite a few years, has watched my personal and professional growth, while encouraging the development of my understanding of neurodiverse relationships.

Have We Gone Nuts?

I also thank God, who keeps me in His safe hands through all my dark hours (and there's been many), leading me through the circumstances and experiences that have allowed me to embark on this journey. After completing my first study, He kept me persisting through the second, to see them to their conclusions and then to authoring this book.

And lastly, but not at all least, I wish to thank all my participants who opened their lives to me with such forthrightness and honesty. They joined with me under a common cause, and willingly shared a part of themselves. Their collaboration, together with, the quality of data their candid input provided and contributions to the survey data, have worked together to give the studies and this associated book, depth and strength of meaning to make these projects the best that they could be.

My aspiration for this book is enhancement of knowledge regarding neurodiverse relationships in the wider community. The hope is that the understanding of those who provide the services, the programs, and the support, will be augmented, so they are better able to accomplish what they do best. The dream is to see an improvement in the lives, and a decline in the challenges faced, of those in neurodiverse relationships around the world.

Notes

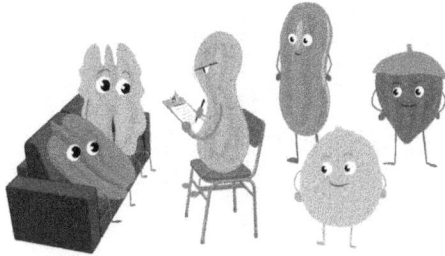

_____

_____

_____

_____

_____

_____

_____

_____

www.ingramcontent.com/pod-product-compliance
Lightning Source LLC
Chambersburg PA
CBHW032050020426

42335CB00011B/269